BABY STEPS

BABY STEPS

HAVING THE CHILD I ALWAYS WANTED
(JUST NOT AS I EXPECTED)

ELISABETH ROHM

WITH EVE ADAMSON

Da Capo
LIFE
LONG

A Member of the Perseus Books Group

Editorial production by *Marra*thon Production Services. www.marrathon.net
Design by Jane Raese
Set in 12.5-point Bulmer

Library of Congress Cataloging-in-Publication Data is available for this book.
ISBN 978-0-7382-1663-8 (hardcover)
ISBN 978-0-7382-1664-5 (e-Book)

First Da Capo Press edition 2013

Published by Da Capo Press
A Member of the Perseus Books Group
www.dacapopress.com

Note: The information in this book is true and complete to the best of our knowledge. This book is intended only as an informative guide for those wishing to know more about health issues. In no way is this book intended to replace, countermand, or conflict with the advice given to you by your own physician. The ultimate decision concerning care should be made between you and your doctor. We strongly recommend you follow his or her advice.

Da Capo Press books are available at special discounts for bulk purchases in the U.S. by corporations, institutions, and other organizations. For more information, please contact the Special Markets Department at the Perseus Books Group, 2300 Chestnut Street, Suite 200, Philadelphia, PA, 19103, or call (800) 810-4145, ext. 5000, or e-mail special.markets@ perseusbooks.com.

10 9 8 7 6 5 4 3 2 1

To my mother, Lisa, and my daughter, Easton,
who opened my heart to love

CONTENTS

My mother always felt like a fish out of water in the South. When she discovered the hippie movement in the 1970s, she was relieved and finally at home. All she ever wanted was to live a creative life as a writer, a simple life without societal pressures. Unfortunately, my father had the exact opposite desire.

My father is German, and his father was a POW in World War II. After the hardship that comes with all of that, my father wanted to live the American dream: success, money, achievement. When he met my mother, he was in New York on a short visa where he was working for a bank, and he passed by a transcendental meditation lecture my mother was guiding on behalf of Maharishi Mahesh Yogi. She had traveled the world with Maharishi since she was eighteen. My father saw her inside and immediately went in and joined the lecture. They started dating and he started meditating. Soon, she accompanied him back to Germany, where I was born.

But although they had that immediate connection, their long-term goals weren't the same. My father, like so many Europeans who grew up during the war, has considered earning a good living an immense priority. There was always that underlying sense of foreboding, like if you didn't work hard enough, you would starve. He has also always been a seeker and a romantic soul who has a mystical, philosophical nature. He loves poetry and opera and the fine arts, and he still meditates, but because he grew up poor and came to the United States to pursue his dream, his outer needs outweighed his inner needs. I sometimes wonder if he would have been someone entirely different if he had not been from Germany and not grown up during the war, but this is who he is. It explains why he was attracted to my mother, and ultimately, it explains why it didn't work. But before it all fell apart, they moved to Westchester County in New York to live the life my father wanted.

Westchester is horse country, with white clapboard houses on rolling green hills, horses grazing in the front yard, and dirt roads along which cars drive at a snail's pace because the most important thing in Westchester is the horses, and a speeding car could spook them. People carve their own pumpkins in Westchester. They use hand-knit napkins for their afternoon tea parties on the terrace or in the rose garden. There is a certain expectation and a certain prestige to Westchester. It's an antiquated place, where those who can afford to live there, who don't want to live in the city and are willing to commute, can live in paradise. It is high-end country living at its best. It is the pages of *Martha Stewart Living* come to life.

My mother identified with some parts of it: the country life, the animals, and especially the flowers. She was a talented gardener, and she made our home beautiful as she struggled to maintain a certain decorum and sense of achievement my father required in order to rise in his profession. They both wanted me to have every advantage as well, and my father believed this was the best place to raise a child. My mother must have agreed, but for her, it was an uncomfortable place, despite the flowers. Her flower-child sensibilities just couldn't relate to the materialism of that life, nor to the sense of achievement so seemingly required. It wasn't her way. She was never a career woman and had no desire to be one. She wasn't interested in status. Her way was to putter in her beautiful garden and live in the moment.

Still, she gave it everything she had. My father needed an ambassador to throw elegant parties for his colleagues when he was a young lawyer, and she did her best, but it was not to be.

I remember the silhouette in the doorway: my father, in his casual weekend clothes, holding a suitcase. My boxer, Romeo, nosed my father's knee and my father petted him firmly, decisively, on the head.

"Don't go," I said. I already knew he would. Both my parents had talked to me about it. But this was Saturday. I didn't get to see my father during the week because he would leave early in the morning and didn't get home until late at night, but on Saturdays, we went riding together. I always looked forward to Saturdays, so how could he be leaving now? The horses would be confused if we didn't show up at the stable. "Don't go," I repeated.

"It's all right," he said. "You'll come visit me next weekend."

As he turned and walked down the drive, I ran to the doorway where he had just been standing, and when he looked back, he must have seen *my* silhouette, clutching each side of the door frame. "Don't go!" I called to him. He just waved and smiled a tight smile. I watched him put his suitcase in the trunk, get in the car, and drive away.

In that moment, I didn't know that I'd ever see him again. Was he gone forever? I sat down on the front step with my chin in my hands and tried to make sense of the brokenhearted feeling I felt welling up: that my father had left and might never come back. And he never did—not to move back in. Once in a while, he would pick me up for the day or the weekend, and I would wait on the front step for him so he didn't have to come into the house, so he and my mother wouldn't argue. I would sprint down the driveway and jump into the backseat of his car and we would do something together, but it was never the same as when he had lived with us and I had been secure in the knowledge that he would always be there.

When I was eight years old, my parents were still "separated" but in couples counseling. My father had moved to the Essex House in New York City. One weekend, when I was staying with him, he had a heart attack on Central Park South. He was taken to the hospital, and when he found out he was going to need open-heart surgery, he thought he might die. My mother came to his bedside, and as is so common during life-threatening situations, truths came out, dirty laundry was aired, and there was no going back. Every relationship has water under the bridge, and in a crisis situation, the levy often breaks. That day marked the real end of their marriage, and he never came back to our home to live with us.

In many relationships that come to an end, there is somebody who is surprised, and somebody with one foot already out the door. My father had one foot out the door, and although he said he wanted to come home, there was no coming home because he was already gone. The writing was already on the wall.

I was emotionally shattered and angry, and I felt betrayed by both of them. Within a year, he had remarried and started another family, and this seemed drastic and cruel from my young vantage point. At the time, I couldn't begin to see my stepmother's beauty, brilliance, or depth. All I knew was that she was taking my father away. I was angry at all of them, but especially my mother and father; my father for leaving, and my mother for being unable to keep him. My father for starting another family I imagined he must love better, because it seemed to me that he chose them over our family. My mother for being so raw, so emotional, so unguarded, and for having no boundaries between us when she was falling apart.

And yet, the responsibility of parenting me and making sure I grew up okay with myself and my life fell almost entirely onto my mother's shoulders. Although I still saw my father and he still helped us out financially, our lifestyle could never equal what it had been before, and my mother had to sacrifice a lot for me. It would be years before she could go her own way.

Until then, my mother wanted to maintain a normal life for me after the divorce. She didn't want to uproot me and take me on some gypsy pilgrimage, like she might have done had she been alone. She understood that I needed to feel safe and secure in my childhood home, so she stayed and struggled to make ends meet, to keep us afloat in the life we'd lived before my father left. It wasn't easy for her.

She could never have made his salary, but she didn't want me to have to pay for their issues. Of course I did—what child of divorce doesn't? But it took me many years to fully acknowledge what my mother gave up, or postponed, for my sake. Now I understand: she could ditch the husband, if necessary (and it did turn out to be necessary), but she had a responsibility to me. I was her child.

Shortly after my father left, she laid it on the line for me:

"Lis, I can't outsmart you. I can't outwit you. I can't spend my days trying to figure out what you're really up to. It's all I can do to keep us going, so you have to make me a deal. If you always tell me the truth, then you will never be punished for what you tell me. But if you don't tell me the truth, there will be consequences for that. Do you understand?"

I did, and I still do. I think a lot of single moms feel like this. Parenting is hard enough in pairs, but when you have to do it on your own, there are limits to what you can realistically tackle. She knew this and right from the start, she demanded honesty. I didn't always give it, but when I didn't, there were consequences, just like she said there would be.

When I was sixteen, my mother allowed me to get a driver's license, with only two conditions.

"If you're drunk, you don't drive," she said. "Just call me and I'll come get you. And don't ever let anyone else drive your car."

So what did I do? I was at a party and I'd had one beer. I thought, *I'll be responsible and I won't drive.* So when my friends and I all went out to buy more beer, I let someone's older brother drive my car. He began to speed down the dark roads in Chappaqua. Then, we crashed head-on into another car.

Amazingly, nobody died, but when my mother went to see the car, she was asked whether anyone survived the accident. The next morning, she took my driver's license and cut it up and threw it away.

"You've lost the right to drive," she said. "And you will not drive again until you can prove that I can trust you again." This is how she always handled things. I lied to her, and I broke her rule, and the consequence was the loss of my driving privileges. She wasn't going to shame me or make me feel like a piece of shit. She was just going to exercise her power to show me that there were repercussions. Which is worse, having a head-on collision or having sex at fourteen? She wouldn't have wished either one of these things on me, but they were decisions I made, situations I got myself into, and there were repercussions in either case. Not shame, but consequences, specifically engineered by her but entirely justified. I could never say that she wasn't fair.

Our history as mother and daughter was long and fraught with turmoil. I didn't make it easy for her to be my mother after my father left. I tortured her, and I tortured him when I saw him, too. I tortured myself. But some objective part of me was always able to stand back and observe the way my mother handled me, and I admired it, even when I was the unwilling recipient of her sense of justice. She was the reason I always knew that I wanted to be a mother. I wanted to be as good at it as she was.

As the next few years passed, my mother and I both struggled, together and separately. Although on the surface we looked like we were maintaining our lifestyle, inside, things were falling apart. Our life was like a beautiful antique dresser: respectable on the outside, but with drawers full of clothes wadded up in balls. Open the drawers and you want to ask, "What's all this shit?" That was us.

She was the one who picked up the pieces after every disappointing interaction I had with my father, when I would come home in tears, but she never shielded me from her pain, emotions, or confusion. Her vulnerability was so raw and out-there for me to see that I could hardly stand it. I wanted to be able to be vulnerable in front of her, but I didn't want her to be vulnerable in front of me. I felt a strong sense of indignation that I had to witness and endure her weakness. I remember one day when I burst into her bedroom to ask what was for dinner, she was sitting on the end of the bed, her bathrobe slipping from her shoulders, her face buried in her hands, weeping. She looked so human and frail, and I hated her for that. I was confused by her humanity. She was supposed to be the one telling *me* that it was time for dinner. Why was she sitting there like that? Why was she crying? Why did I have to see it? The picture is burned in my memory.

She never hid her tears from me, whether she cried because all the bills were late and the check from my father still hadn't arrived, or because she felt like an alien in a place she never would have chosen for herself, or out of frustration at my behavior—my anger and refusal to participate in my classes at school. Sometimes it made me so uncomfortable that I vowed never to cry in front of my own child. I hated that I sometimes had to be the one to say, "Mom, the house is a mess," or "Mom, we need to eat dinner now," or "Mom, I have a doctor's appointment today. You have to take me there and we have to be on time."

Who are we supposed to be in front of each other? Are we allowed to be human in front of our daughters? In front of our mothers? Or are we supposed to pretend to be strong because the world expects it, even while we are crumbling inside? I honestly don't know the answer to that one yet.

Maybe she should have shielded me more, but she simply didn't know how. My mother was who she was. Between the two of us, there were no boundaries. My rage and her vulnerability clashed in ways that seemed more extreme than they would have if our family had remained whole, but at least I always knew she was on my side. Painful as it was to see my mother struggling rather than putting up a front of strength and impenetrability, I understood that she didn't want any smoke and mirrors in our relationship. She wanted me to learn how to be an honest person, who not only knows how to tell the truth to others, but who can tell the truth to herself. To me, it was sometimes too much honesty, but it also worked. I have grown into a brutally honest person. Sometimes that has served me well, and sometimes there have been casualties.

But at the time, I was the casualty. At fourteen, I was so academically out of whack the public school system labeled me as "impossible to educate."

I think if you are a smart kid, you tend to go out to the edge and look over to see how far you will fall if you jump off. Just because you're curious. Or because you're angry enough to really do it. Any parent with a smart and curious kid is going to have her hands full. For me, working that edge was about refusing to do homework, refusing to participate in class, and refusing to be part of the system.

They called it "going on strike," and it took the public school system two years to determine that I did not have a learning disability, that I did not have ADHD, that I was not mentally ill, but that I was simply angry, messed up, and incorrigible. I was the kid who ended up at that lone desk out in the hall. I was in the "learning disabled" classes with all the other kids who couldn't seem to make it in the system or refused to try. I'd had my brain tested and retested, my IQ tested, my stress level tested by how tightly I gripped a pencil during a test. I'd taken handwriting tests and psychological tests and stared at shapes and geometrical patterns, and I'd spent countless hours with the school counselor. When they at last offically pronounced me extremely smart but extremely angry and hurt, they said I needed to be in a place where I could get the attention I was lacking. They said I was acting out from an emotional place, and they were not equipped to handle that. They said I was out. The last two weeks of middle school, I was not allowed to go back on school grounds.

My mother did everything she could to give me the tools to deal with our family trauma and my own anger. I'd been in therapy since I was eight years old, even before the divorce, to help me deal with the verbal violence I witnessed regularly from my parents and the gradual disintegration of our family unit. I'd spent years attending an ashram in upstate New York with my mother—it was my summer camp—wearing saris and participating in rituals and attending self-help programs, first for kids and eventually, for teens. But the simple fact was that her efforts to "fix" me weren't working, according to the system. I was failing every single class. I wasn't making it. I was *choosing* not to make it. That was the final determination.

I remember the moment when I asked my shrink if I could read the court-ordered analysis that the public school required in order to boot me out. He should never have let me read it, but I did. It contained everything, every gory detail of my past and my parents' breakup, including details I didn't even know or remember. It was a *War of the Roses* story, full of volatility and emotional violence, and it had my mother written all over it: unchecked expression spewed across the pages, my mother imposing her experience on me yet again, making it mine instead of allowing me to have my own. And the details—details that painted a picture far more difficult than I'd imagined. Details of private things that government officials and school officials had now read: exhaustive accounts of my parents' fights, my embarrassing reactions to their fights and their therapy, and some things I barely believed could be true. I could feel the tension building inside of me as I read, until finally I threw the papers onto the floor, climbed up on the couch, and screamed at the top of my lungs:

"You liar! I hate you! I hate you all!"

Then I collapsed on the floor and wept. It wasn't my best moment. My heart had been broken into a million pieces. It was quite a display, I'm sure, but my emotions were true and I couldn't argue with their final verdict: I didn't fit in. I was too damaged. I was too "complicated." They could not educate me. I needed more than they could give. A judge had ordered it: I was done.

When I recovered and my mother came to take me home, we had a serious discussion. She didn't judge me. She didn't shame me. In fact, she understood completely, and she probably felt responsible. But I was still years from graduation, so I had two options. I could drop out, take my GED, and we could travel the world together. "The world would be your classroom," she told me. "But I need to be honest with you. For the rest of your life, you'll always know you didn't finish high school, and people will judge you because of that. You'll always be like an outsider looking in. You'll always know you gave up."

Or, she told me, I could go to private school.

The problem with private school was that, based on my academic record, the only schools likely to accept me were schools for juvenile delinquents. There were options. We browsed them and visited several. There was the posh $16,000-a-year school for rich kids who didn't feel like fitting in, but we both knew we could never afford that kind of tuition. There was the state-funded school, but it looked more like a prison than a school, and the description scared us both. We finally settled on a school in upstate New York that seemed like the perfect compromise; some court-ordered kids were there, but others at the school just didn't fit in for one reason or another. It was affordable, but not scary, or so we thought. Best of all, I would escape my life thus far and get out into the world, where I could become my own person. I would leave home, and I would never move back. I was fourteen years old.

*T*o people who aren't actors, acting may not seem like a way to discover the truth about yourself and your place in the world. It may not seem like a way to stay grounded. It may seem more like make-believe, or living your life as someone else. But for me, acting has been my center and the thing that always brings me back to myself.

Through acting, I worked out my issues about love. Through acting, I found lovers and father figures, friends and mother figures, and a whole slew of mentors who played various roles in my life—brothers, uncles, even children. Acting grew me from a girl to a woman, from a partner to a mother. It has been alchemical in my life. It has established rules for my life that I have lived by, and they have worked for me, even when I broke them. Acting has been the law of my land.

Of course, that hasn't always been the case. In fact, I never even wanted to be an actor.

My first acting role was at Sarah Lawrence College. After high school, I decided to attend Sarah Lawrence, not just because my mother had gone there but because it's known to be a great school for writers, and that's what I wanted to be. A writer. I dreamed about it. I was passionate about it. I imagined myself as an intellectual, producing great novels that would change lives. My mother had always wanted to be a writer, but she hadn't been successful or made any money at it. I would fulfill her unfulfilled dream, but not just because it was her dream. It was my dream, too. It's how I imagined my future life. For me, it was the obvious choice.

Once I was in college, however, I found myself in a dormitory full of theater majors. I thought of myself as intellectual and bookish, and I was surprised and charmed by this group of loud, vibrant, dynamic circus people who loved to express themselves. Meeting them planted a seed in me. I wanted to join the circus, too. I was drawn to them because of their openness, although I felt like they were very different from me because I intellectualized everything and tried to feel my feelings as little as possible.

Being a college student, I was also a little bit boy crazy, and there were some cute theater guys who caught my eye. One of them was a boy named Eric Mabius (who later went on to star in many movies and TV shows), who was handsome and open-hearted, and I found myself imagining what it might be like to be in a play, too—a play with *him.* I had a crush on him, and I thought that we would end up together in the cast of some play or another. The idea unnerved me but interested me. On a whim, in a moment of sudden courage, I decided I would audition for the next play that came along. Maybe Eric, or some other cute guy, would audition, too. If nothing else, all those wonderful circus people might start to see me as one of them.

I didn't know anything about the play I auditioned for. It was called *Bondage,* by David Henry Hwang, and not only did that cute Eric *not* audition for it, but I got the lead role. As the dominatrix. With the leather and the mask and the whip.

Wait a minute, I thought. I wasn't ready for something this . . . committed. I was just trying to get some attention, maybe a date. I hadn't really thought about being in a play, in front of a whole audience full of people, especially playing a character like this. A dominatrix? I was from *Westchester,* for God's sake! What was I thinking? The whole idea seemed ridiculous.

But there I was on the cast list:

TERRI: Elisabeth Rohm

I read the script. It made me even more nervous. Sadomasochism, racism, intimacy, sex . . . this was heavy stuff. Who did I think I was? I couldn't exactly quit, but maybe I could get fired. When we started rehearsals, I decided I just wouldn't get into it. I spoke my lines without feeling. I was inhibited in my movements. I was *embarrassed.* I was phoning it in because why the hell would I want anybody to associate me with that character anyway? I feared I'd get a reputation. "Ooh, Elisabeth Rohm . . . the *dominatrix.*" I blushed just thinking about it.

Apparently, my displeasure was pretty obvious, and the director of the play complained to the head of the theater department, an amazing woman named Shirley Kaplan. Shirley called me into the office shortly after rehearsals had begun and sat me down and told me the director wanted to replace me. I remember feeling both relieved and offended. It was what I'd hoped for, but still . . .

"Lis, here's the deal," she said. "Maybe you're fine with being replaced. Maybe you don't want to play this part at all. But before you decide, let me just ask you this. What's standing in your way?"

I thought about that for a minute. My pride wouldn't let me say, "Well, I was hoping this one cute boy named Eric might be in the play," or "I didn't have any idea what the play was about." But the real truth was that I feared I couldn't do it. I didn't know how to become a character. I had no idea what I was doing. Most of all, I didn't *want* to become a character like *that.*

"I guess . . . I just don't like the character," I said. It was true. I thought the character was slutty. I didn't want people to think *I* was slutty. My inability to play the part well was my way of proving that I had nothing to do with that character.

"Do what you need to do," she said, "but let me tell you this. If you want to be an actor, you need to understand that acting is not about judging. You have to find the humanity in every character. You have to find their point of view, and it's very seldom that anyone thinks that they themselves are a monster or a slut or even a bad person. You have to find out why the character does what she does, why she lives the way she lives. That's the whole point of acting. That's your job, to get in there and understand her. It doesn't mean you become her. It just means you find empathy, and common ground."

I'd never really thought about any of this before, especially since I had no intention of becoming an actor. But her philosophic approach intrigued me. If acting really was about understanding people and analyzing human behavior, that sounded pretty interesting. It was an intellectual approach I could relate to. I'd even considered psychology as a profession, and I also wanted to be a more empathetic person, because empathy was a quality my mother had, and always valued in others. This acting thing might be good for me.

I thought about the famous actors I knew about, and even my theater friends. Did I associate them with the roles they played? Sometimes, but not in a bad way. I admired the ones who could transform themselves and portray the humanity in any character. Unexpectedly, this sounded like something worth pursuing.

This was the first time I began to conceptualize the idea of a rule or a *law* related to acting. Before, it had seemed like it was all fun and games and flirting and make-believe, without structure or purpose, but the fact that there were rules and techniques to this art form appealed to me. After my crazy hippie childhood so void of conventional boundaries, I liked the idea of an artistic life, but I also craved structure. With acting, I began to see, I could be free and wild and also safe. A play wasn't real life. It had a finite ending. If I could *love* the dominatrix, if I could find common ground, maybe I could actually be good at *playing* her without having to *be* her, without being threatened by her. I began to change my mind about the character of Terri. She wasn't dangerous after all. She was an exercise in empathy.

I didn't quit. I powered through the show, I got better, and then we opened, and I discovered something else unexpected and magical about the theater. Before I went on stage, I had the worst stage fright. I was terrified. I remember reminding myself to breathe, breathe, breathe!

Then I went out there in my leather and my mask, brandishing my whip, and I did it. I performed the hell out of that part. It was like an out-of-body experience. All my pent-up emotion, all my unrealized passion, all my anxiety and doubt about myself and my life transformed into the passion, anxiety, and doubt in the character. I was standing up there in the dark in front of hundreds of people, powerful and vulnerable and overcoming all my fear. It was the most incredible feeling I'd ever had.

I remember during one scene, I had my leg up on a block and I was wearing these patent-leather high-heeled boots and cracking the whip and I was thinking, *This is exactly what I didn't want to do, and here I am doing it.* I could hardly believe it was me. I felt so courageous! At the end of the show, my character sits down and takes off her mask because she decides she needs love and she wants to have a real relationship with the man in the play. She's through with role-playing. She wants him to know who she really is. This, I completely understood. When I took off that mask onstage on that night, it was me, taking off the mask of who I thought I should be and exposing who I really was to a room full of people I'd never even met.

It was the highest I'd ever felt, and considering I was in college, I'd felt pretty high already on occasion. I became the dominatrix, and yet I was completely Lis. And then it was over, and I remember the applause and the energy from the audience rolling over me like a wave of love.

I was hooked. It was such a rush, and I was addicted. Acting wasn't just about getting attention (although I realized that I actually enjoyed that). It was also about revealing myself. It was a lesson in *me*. What had started as a ploy to meet a boy turned into an intellectual quest and then finally became visceral and passionate and transformative, and I couldn't get enough.

I began to change my plans. Writing, in many ways, was the same as acting, I realized. It had the same goal, but the medium was different. The more I acted and wrote, the more I realized that maybe I was a better actor than a writer. When I was about to graduate, I decided to give it a try. Acting. Why not?

"Lis, are you sure you want to do this?" my mother said to me over the phone. "I don't want you to be disillusioned. Acting is such a competitive career. I want you to be happy."

I understood her fear. She'd always dreamed of becoming a successful artist, and her dreams had been dashed, but I had a trick up my sleeve. What seemed to my mother a precarious and risky choice was actually a safe choice for me. My dreams couldn't be dashed, because acting wasn't my dream. It was more like an experiment. It was fun, I enjoyed it, it did something for me, but I wasn't emotionally invested. It was still relatively new to me and I wanted more time with it, but I wasn't necessarily committed to it as a career choice. My dream had always been to be a writer. If I tried *that* and failed, I truly would have been disillusioned. Instead, I played it safe. If acting didn't work out, I would just do something else. It was a little like deciding to marry your best friend instead of the guy you are head-over-heels about because you know you'll stay saner. It wasn't a passionate decision. It was logical.

Maybe that's why it worked out so well.

After college, I got a job working for an agent in New York, and through a series of lucky coincidences and friends of friends, got a meeting with soap opera goddess and writer Claire Labine.

Claire and I connected immediately, like mother and daughter. After we met, she wrote me a three-year contract and a role on *One Life to Live*. She was in the process of adding some new characters on the show, and I was part of a father-daughter team. My character was named Dorothy, the estranged daughter of an alcoholic journalist. Dorothy had a sad, tragic story about losing her mother, having an abortion, and having father issues she wanted to heal.

Hmm, that sounded familiar. And what I found, when I played Dorothy working out her issues, was that it was like I was actually working out my own issues right there on camera. Dorothy's truth was like my truth.

I had never imagined myself on a soap opera. I had bigger aspirations, but to get a job like this so quickly after college felt like a major victory. At first, working on a soap opera was nerve-wracking. It's not like a movie, where you do every scene five thousand times at every single angle—from the air, from the side, from underneath, from the right, and from the left. We were lucky if we got to rehearse a scene twice before the cameras were rolling, and then we were filming, one shot, all the way to the end of the scene. It was similar to theater, where you have to keep going even if you make a mistake. It reminds me of that Martha Graham quote: "Artists take leap after leap in the dark." That's what it felt like. Whenever I reached the end of a scene, I would have this feeling of elation: "I did it! I didn't crash and burn! Maybe I could do better next time, but at least I didn't screw it up!"

We would do an entire episode every day, sometimes more. It all moved very quickly and we had to learn a lot of material, so it was great training. It also felt structured. I liked that. There were unwritten laws governing the running of a soap opera. We did the same thing every day, and I loved that I could be the free-spirited artist but also work within the structure of the show. There was no time for endless rehearsal or waiting for "inspiration." On a production schedule like that, everybody has to get the job done. I worked hard, I learned fast, and I got paid. I felt like the luckiest girl in the world.

But six months later, the story line wasn't popular enough in the ratings. Claire got sacked and so did everyone associated with the new story line. It was my first big professional failure, and I was stunned. Fired? How could I be fired? I had a three-year contract!

But it was over. I remember walking down the hallway, weeping openly. How could they do this to me? How could they cut Dorothy loose? Was my dream of being an actor dead already, after such a promising beginning?

One of the divas on the show saw me and pulled me into her dressing room.

"I don't know why you're crying," she said sternly. "Everyone who gets fired from this place becomes a huge star. Judith Light was fired from here. Tommy Lee Jones was fired from here. You should consider yourself fortunate."

I didn't know if what she said was true or not, but misery loves company, and it did make me feel better. Judith Light? Tommy Lee Jones? I swallowed. Maybe she was right. I wallowed in self-pity for about five minutes. Then I shook it off and decided that I would become as famous as Tommy Lee Jones.

After that little setback, I decided to treat acting like a business. I didn't like the randomness of my dismissal, so I decided to impose a structure on my pursuit of acting. I would follow certain rules. I would audition religiously. I would learn everything I could about the industry. And every Saturday night, I would write letters to producers, directors, actors, everyone who really inspired me to be an actor. Based on those letters, I got meetings with Kevin Costner, Paula Wagner, who produced *Mission Impossible* with Tom Cruise, and Jim Sheridan, who directed *My Left Foot*. I felt like I was making progress. Even my mother began to recant her doubts.

"You're really taking this acting seriously," she said. "I'm impressed with how organized you are. And ambitious. You might really get somewhere with this."

My stepmother Jessica, who is a brilliant businesswoman, was a great cheerleader for me, too, and totally saw my vision.

I decided to spend more time in Los Angeles, because that's where it was all happening. As much as I loved New York, I realized this was a necessary transition, so I relocated, and nobody could dampen my confidence. As soon as I arrived in LA, I made an appointment with an entertainment lawyer, marched into his office with a portfolio filled with all the clips of interviews I'd done while on *One Life to Live,* and dropped them on his desk. I said, "Here's my scrapbook of interviews. I'm going to be a big star, so get ready."

He just looked at me, probably wondering who the hell I thought I was. "Sure, kid," he said. Five days later, I auditioned for a pilot for *The Invisible Man,* starring Kyle MacLachlan, produced by Dick Wolf, and I got the part! I called my entertainment lawyer, and with more than a little attitude, I told him, "Negotiate my pilot. Told ya so."

I was ecstatic. Five days in LA, and already, a TV pilot? We filmed the pilot and I felt so important being involved in the project. Then Dick Wolf called me.

"Well, kiddo, it's just not going to work out." He was telling me the pilot didn't get picked up and wouldn't be produced as a TV show. I was devastated. "Unfortunately, it was an expensive project, but it just wasn't all there," he said.

My next thought was about Dick Wolf.

"Oh my God," I said. "I'm nobody, but everybody knows you. Is this a big deal for your career? Are you going to be okay?"

I'll never forget what he said to me.

"Next."

"What?" I said.

"Next. That's my philosophy about failures. 'Next.'"

I got it. I don't think I've ever internalized a loss or a failure for very long, no matter how big or small, because of that conversation. I hear his voice in my head saying, *Next.* He made the loss of that pilot seem so unimportant, when he was the one who had risked so much. I've always admired him for being able to have that kind of perspective.

Back then, it was harder for me. I saw this as a step backward, and I began to reconsider my choices, and my move to LA. I even toyed with the idea of quitting acting altogether, but until I knew for sure, I decided to keep auditioning. Then I got a screen test for Barry Levinson, and an audition for Michael Apted, who was casting for the James Bond film *The World Is Not Enough.* Better yet, I was flown to London for a screen test.

In London, I met casting directors Roz and John Hubbard. They told me that if I didn't get the Bond film, they wanted to cast me in a BBC miniseries they were doing. Despite my high hopes, I didn't get the film. They cast Denise Richards instead. But I did get the BBC miniseries. It was called *Eureka Street.* And off I went to Ireland for five months.

On *Eureka Street,* I played a young woman named Max who grew up in Ireland, and whose father was the American ambassador who had just been killed. Like my character on *One Life to Live,* this character had a lot of father issues. She was a rich American girl who was suddenly on her own. I could totally relate to this part. My father was very much alive, but I still felt the sting of his absence. Playing Max helped me to understand even more about how abandoned I felt. Max and I had similar trust issues and intimacy issues, and at the end of the show, when she marries the person she loves and finally opens her heart and feels love again, I felt hope that maybe this would happen for me, too. I found myself in Max, and I hoped I could find some of Max in me.

As I was navigating the early years of my career, I was also always looking for love, hoping with every new role and every new move that I might meet someone right for me. Yet somehow, the relationships never worked out. During *Eureka Street,* I dated an actor on the show named Vincent, but after the filming was over, I went back to the States to audition for a new spin-off of *Buffy the Vampire Slayer* called *Angel,* and we quickly realized a long-distance relationship wasn't going to work. I wasn't going to go back to Ireland, and he wasn't going to come to LA. As much as I wanted love, in reality, I was still too career driven to make any sacrifices for it. Vincent and I parted ways. Sometimes I dreamed about the perfect man, the perfect family, becoming a mother, but it all seemed theoretical and far away. It wouldn't be Vincent.

My audition for *Angel* in front of Joss Whedon and David Greenwalt was a good one (I even threw a chair!). I think they liked that I was a little bit off-kilter. I liked how dark the character was, but when they offered me the part, I had second thoughts. I'd just done a BBC miniseries and I'd been screen testing for movies—did I really want to do a *Buffy* spinoff? Was that the direction for me? I remember getting on the phone with Joss Whedon and talking about the importance of exploring the themes of good and evil and the power they have in our lives. I wanted to do serious work, not a vampire show, but the more we talked, the more Joss convinced me that although the show seemed campy, there were serious undertones and messages in every episode. I said yes to *Angel* and to playing the part of Detective Kate Lockley.

Kate also had intimacy issues. Her father was the chief of police and he treated her like one of the boys. She longed for a more meaningful relationship with him. I began to wonder why I kept getting roles with daddy issues! Was I wearing some psychic sign that revealed how much I knew about this subject? There must have been a reason why I was finding myself over and over again in every character I played.

Kate and her father had some scenes that helped me understand how I blamed my father for not giving me love in exactly the way I wanted. I realized that a child's view of the parent isn't necessarily based in reality. It is heightened and sensitive and vulnerable, and things are bigger to a child than they are to an adult. I began to see all that through Kate. As Kate, I had to listen to my father's feelings and deal with them, and it was like hearing my own father talking to me. It changed me. I began to wonder if I could forgive him. Maybe he could forgive me, too. I'm sure having me for a daughter wasn't easy.

I was on *Angel* for two seasons, and I loved being on the show, but ever since filming the pilot for *The Invisible Man,* I had stayed in touch with Dick Wolf in hopes of getting involved with one of his projects. I think he's brilliant and I wanted to audition for everything he ever did. When I found out there was an available part on *Law & Order,* I jumped at it. This was one of the most successful television series of all time. And my father was a lawyer! I was *made* for that show! I showed up for the audition full of confidence.

I didn't count on Angie Harmon. I'll never forget seeing her in the parking lot for the first time. She wore a white silk blouse and she had a much fuller, more grown-up figure than I did. Her long black hair glistened. I remember noticing her breasts, then looking down at mine unhappily. There was no comparison. She was a goddess. I had big hips and no boobs and I definitely didn't have cheekbones like hers, but I sucked it up and went inside and gave it all I could. Never mind that I still looked like a round-cheeked little cherub compared to Angie. When she got the part instead of me, I was devastated. I couldn't understand it. Didn't they realize my father was an attorney? What did they care about chiseled cheekbones! I actually know about the law! And wasn't she *too* beautiful for that part? She's the kind of woman who could cause a car crash just walking down the street. I was cute, but not hot. Isn't that more appropriate for a lawyer?

No matter how many reasons I concocted for why they should have hired me for the role, the fact remained that I was out and Angie was in. I was disappointed, but I persevered. A few months later, I got a role on *Bull,* a new series about stockbrokers and their lives. I played Alison Jeffers, opposite Stanley Tucci, with a wonderful cast of actors and a staff of excellent writers.

This was one of the most exciting times in my career because I was double dipping—running from the set of *Angel* to the set of *Bull* and back again. Unfortunately, *Bull* didn't last. This was before the stock market crash and Enron and Martha Stewart and all of that. If it had come a little later, I think it would have lasted longer. It was cancelled in the middle of the first season, which crushed all of us in the cast because we knew what a great show it was.

Every time something in my career fell apart, I considered quitting acting. Every time, I told myself that I never really wanted to be an actor anyway, so this was my chance to go do something else. I almost changed career course after *Bull* was cancelled. Then Angie Harmon decided to quit *Law & Order.* I found out about this from a publicist friend of mine named Karen Tencer. She told me to call Dick Wolf and ask for an audition. My ego was still bruised and I didn't want to call him, but she talked me into it. When he said no, that I wasn't right for the part, I told Karen what he said, and she told me to argue with him, to keep calling, to insist on an audition. "Your agents are never going to fight for you as much as you will fight for yourself," she said. I called him back. Finally, he agreed to let me audition.

This time, I wasn't sure at all that I would get the part, and as I auditioned, I felt like they weren't leaning toward me for the role at all. Still, I gave it everything I had.

I was driving along the Pacific Coast Highway the day I got the call from Dick Wolf.

"You got it, Lis."

"What?"

I got it. I got it? All I could hear was the crashing of the Pacific Ocean in my right ear, and the good news echoing in my left ear. I'd done it! I'd gotten a part on *Law & Order*, one of the most well-known and widely watched television dramas of all time, and the legendary Dick Wolf was calling me personally to tell me that I was going to play Assistant DA Serena Southerlyn.

"You're going to love me and hate me," he said.

"No!" I protested. "I only love you!"

"You have to leave for New York in seventy-two hours," he said. "So start packing, kiddo."

"I'm ready!" I said, already planning what to pack in the back of my mind. "Thank you, thank you!"

"You have no idea what you're getting into," he said. "It's a golden cage."

I didn't know what he meant at the time, but I found out later it was true. All I knew was that I had attained something I had busted my butt to get, and I was on my way. I'll never forget the feeling of landing very late at night at JFK with my cat and seven suitcases. I had come home. After all that time in California, with its ups and downs, highs and lows, I felt like I had finally returned to a safe place I totally understood. New York has always been the only place I call home, even after all these years of living in La La Land. It's the place where I feel most like myself, and now I was about to play a part that was smack in the middle of my comfort zone.

After years of playing characters with emotional issues like mine, it was a relief to play someone on a show that was plot driven rather than character driven. The show was about the story, not about me or any of the regular characters. A television series was steady—especially one this well established. I liked that idea very much. That night, a driver took me to my new corporate housing where I would live for three months while I acclimated to the ten- to fourteen-hour-a-day shooting schedule. In the spring of 2001, Serena Southerlyn had arrived in New York, and my life would never be the same.

My first day on the set, Angie Harmon was there. She put her arm around me and gave me the tour with a huge smile on her face, giddy with joy that she was leaving. I was slightly overwhelmed by her happiness, and hugely curious about it. I was thinking, *Thank God she quit!* But here she was, obviously overjoyed to be leaving. I didn't know why. I couldn't imagine why she would want to leave. To me, such a role was a dream come true, but I wasn't going to ask any questions. She'd opened the door of the golden cage for me. She was out, and I was in. She was happy, I was happy, so what did it matter why?

Walking down the hallway with Dick Wolf to shoot my very first scene with Sam Waterston, I had a lump the size of a fist in my throat. I didn't think I'd be able to get my lines out. I could barely speak. I was paralyzed with nerves. I was an experienced actor by now, but this was the biggest job I'd ever been given. In that first scene, all I had to do was stand in a hallway, take law books from a dolly, and put them on a shelf. How hard could it be? That's what I was thinking: *Just put the books on the shelf, Lis.* Sam Waterston approached me and said something about the case, "Blah blah blah," and I said something back, "Blah blah blah" (that's how it felt!), and that was it. I was so incredibly grateful that my first scene was such a short one. I felt like I had that lump in my throat for a week.

Being on *Law & Order* is all consuming. It was a hulking, massive experience. It became my life. My life became law, and there was no breaking this law. After years of metaphorical lawlessness, I was about to learn exactly what it was like to exist within the intricate structure of a legal drama.

I loved this time in my life. It was intense and fulfilling and it galvanized my lifelong love of being on television. I had to fall in love with *Law & Order* before I could want to leave it for other creative endeavors. It was a very long time before I understood why Angie Harmon was ready to leave. I was too busy falling in love. *Law & Order* was my new romance, my grand passion.

Law & Order was and is a quintessentially New York show. People often stopped to tell me that we had filmed an episode where they worked or near where they lived. People also liked to tell me how much they loved Sam Waterston. When I walked down the street with Sam, people would stop and stare or crowd around him like he was one of the Beatles.

It wasn't at all like filming a show in LA, where you drive in a cart onto the Paramount lot and you get a spacious trailer and you smell the sea breeze and flowers whenever you step outside. Dick Wolf had taken over a warehouse on the Hudson River and turned it into the *Law & Order* studio, so we smelled the river and the city every day. We smelled mold and rotting fish. Filming *Law & Order* was gritty. We were working stiffs, real New Yorkers, and every day, we went to work like everyone else in the city.

I had a view of the river from my small dressing room. The whole building was musty and sometimes buggy. It was dark and moody and intellectual. It was the best place I could imagine. I built a family there. It was my new circus. Nothing felt as good as stepping out onto that darkened stage every day, ready to film.

I liked my character, too. Serena Southerlyn was a do-gooder. She would defend any downtrodden person who came along, which didn't always work for the prosecutor's office. She couldn't just fight the case objectively. She was a humanitarian, and she would have probably made a better public defender. I admired that about her.

Most of all, I admired my fellow actors, especially Sam, who became like a father to me. In the past, some of the female characters had romantic tension with Sam, but my character saw him as more of a mentor, and that's how I felt personally, too. Sam and Fred Thompson, who also became near and dear to me, taught me what it meant to take acting seriously. They treated the job like any other job that requires you to be prompt and come prepared and not waste anybody's time—like construction work or food service or stepping onto the line every day. Sam and Fred had this work ethic that we were all in this together and we all shared in the toil. The rest of the people on the show also became like family. Diane Wiest was divine, her distinctive laugh and warm energy a highlight on the set. And who could forget Jerry Orbach, one of the most gracious and loving people I've ever met?

When I first joined *Law & Order,* during the very first week, I threw a big party for myself to celebrate. I invited everybody in the whole cast, and the only people who showed up were Jerry Orbach and his wife, Elaine. They stayed for a whole hour. Jerry taught me that when you are part of something, you act like you are part of it. There is no need to act cool, or better than everybody else. When you are part of the circus, you participate in the circus. You don't ignore the clowns, or the trapeze artists. You are all one big family, and there is a strong sense of family values.

As much as I thrived on the dark, gritty intellect of the show, apparently I stood out a bit from the traditional characters, or so everybody liked to talk about in the press. I was the first blonde they had ever hired on *Law & Order* and there were a lot of hurtful comments out there about me, comparing me to the other women on the show. I learned to stop reading what people published about me because it made me feel terrible. "She's blond, she shouldn't be on the show, she doesn't look like a lawyer, she's not like the others, she's different, different, different." My whole life I'd been hearing how *different* I was, when all I wanted was to be like everyone else. I was tempted to dye my hair brown, just so I wouldn't stand out so much.

I finally decided my difference could be a gift to the show. I became known for my blond hair and Diet-Coke habit on the set, and I did my best to brighten up the place. I decorated my dressing room like a Ralph Lauren studio, with red walls and equestrian paintings and a celery-green chaise longue with curves like a woman. I invited people into my dressing room to sit in the leather chairs and visit, or thumb through the law books that I kept on a shelf but never needed to read because Sam was such a bastion of legal knowledge.

My days were all about the schedule. This was a typical day on the set: A driver named Carlos would pick me up at five in the morning and take me to the studio on Hudson River Parkway. I would get there around six and go straight into hair and makeup. They would throw a few newspapers at us if we wanted them, and I had to try very hard not to annoy anybody by talking too much at such an early hour about my twenty-something adventures in New York City (dates gone wrong or right, red carpet events, parties, romantic entanglements—it was a busy and exciting time).

At around seven, we would go into rehearsal. We would rehearse the first scene, talk about it, block it, and then leave to get dressed while they lit the scene. This is when people started to wake up and talk to each other. We might hear Frank Sinatra blasting out of Dennis Farina's dressing room during the time he was on the show, or in Jerry Orbach's time, we would peek inside his dressing room to see what interesting thing he might be doing. Dianne Wiest was always laughing, and we could all hear the sweet soothing sound of her voice down the hall. Fred Thompson's door was always wide open. Anybody was welcome to come in and see what he was up to—usually reading something political, perhaps plotting his presidential campaign. He was brilliant, but also so human that you would never know how distinguished he was. Fred was surprisingly user-friendly. He always made himself accessible and he made everybody feel like they were just as smart as he was, even though he is a genius. You would never know you were involved with anyone who had any influence over Supreme Court decisions, or who was a potential US president, because he seemed like such a regular guy.

While we were all in hair and makeup, we would sit around on our breaks and debate and say smart things. At least, they would say smart things! There was always this pressure to be in the know on that show, because you can't sit in a room with Sam Waterston and Dick Wolf and Fred Thompson and not have something intelligent to say. There was a lot of pressure on that set to prove oneself, and that worked for me. It's one of the things I miss most about that show. A lot of movies and television shows are fun, but not necessarily intellectual. *Law & Order* was rare in that way.

After we were dressed, we would go back to the set and film the first scene. That's how the rest of the day would go—rehearse, dress while they lit the scene, shoot the scene. Sam Waterston and I would have lunch together. We would order vegan food and I would end my meal with a vegan chocolate cupcake. In the afternoons, we would meet to discuss the script for the next week, and then we would keep filming. We were usually out by eight to ten at night.

Over the course of five years, I transformed from a round-faced little girl with a blond bob to a more curvaceous, small-waisted, deeper-voiced grown woman with long blond hair. I grew up as Serena Southerlyn. We grew up together. When you play a character over the course of years, you can become indistinguishable. The show and

Serena became part of me. *Law & Order* changed me, but I did my fair share of changing *Law & Order*, too.

When I came on the show, I was appalled at the Amish-looking, stiff gray suits we were supposed to wear. All the women were dressed down to look sexless and androgynous, their natural beauty stifled, and I wasn't interested in that at all. They would show me these suits I had to wear, and I would say, "No way, I am not wearing that." I would wear red lipstick, and they would tell me that a lawyer wouldn't wear red lipstick. The weekend I got my bangs cut, you would have thought I'd chopped off my own head. The entire production team was in an uproar. *Bangs? A lawyer wouldn't wear bangs! Cute blond bangs? Call the Marines! She cut her bangs!* Were they worried the show would be cancelled because Serena Southerlyn had *bangs?* I was pretty sure the show would be just fine.

I've always believed that a smart woman can still be sexy. Sarah Lawrence was filled with smart sexy women, and my stepmother embodied this principle. I grew up assuming that you could wear stiletto heels and a fitted Gucci suit and still be brilliant—in fact, you might even be more effective and powerful. I didn't understand why we had to be dressed down or made dowdy to be believable as lawyers.

By the end of my time there, the producers had gradually conceded my point. I gave a little; they gave a little. I felt like I brought some light to those dank dressing rooms. I insisted on being happy and the golden cage Dick had warned me about actually felt safe. I've never been afraid to live the off-kilter life of an actor, but of all the jobs I could have gotten in the context of the bohemian career I'd chosen, this had to be the least bohemian of them all. I began to feel balanced, even as part of me wanted to throw myself off balance again.

But as much as I gained, I also lost. Being in *Law & Order* left little time for anything or anyone else. None of my relationships lasted. They all imploded because the show was my priority, because I wasn't

ally hung in there. During vulnerable times, it's easy to fall prey to that inner monologue we always have going on in our heads that convinces us how wronged we are. Thank goodness nobody could hear mine.

I'm sure Ron also felt the immense pressure we were under to succeed because we had spent such a large sum of money on this gamble, and he had absolutely no control over the results. It was strange to be so let down and also so hopeful at the same time, but we persevered. Every time I got another shot, I imagined that we were rolling the dice, just like everyone else doing IVF all over the world, powerless to control the result. It felt like those shots contained a magic potion. If it was swirled together in just the right way and injected into me with a needle, I would have a baby. If it was swirled together in the wrong direction, if the angle of the needle was wrong, or we injected at the wrong time of day, or I was in the wrong mood at the moment of injection, then that baby would evaporate into the ether.

Dr. Sahakian regularly monitored the development of my eggs with an imaging machine, which allowed him to look at my ovaries, count the follicles that contained the eggs, and monitor the development of the follicles into fat little pods that could rupture and produce a ready-and-willing egg. After the first look inside at my ovaries after being on the stimulating drugs for a few weeks, he noticed that one of them was flattened and not producing many eggs at all.

"It's weird," he said. "Your ovary on the left side is flat, with no good follicles. The other side has a few good ones, though. Let's just stay on the drugs a little bit longer."

My first thought was, *the abortion*. Had they done something wrong during that abortion all those years ago? Had they destroyed one of my ovaries? Was that the whole problem? I was wracked with guilt. I asked Dr. Sahakian if that could be the reason.

"Who knows?" he said. "But we're here now, so the reason doesn't matter."

It mattered to me. Who has a flattened ovary? I kept thinking someone had to have done that to me, but I'll probably never know the answer.

Dr. Sahakian said the other ovary looked good with viable follicles, and the drugs would help those eggs to continue to mature and get juicy (as he put it). Throughout the visits, he continued to watch the follicles. They weren't developing quite as quickly as he liked, so he had me do another round of the drugs before retrieving the eggs for the fertilization procedure. I worried that this meant it might not work.

But on August 4, we began the HCG injections, which stimulate egg development, and then we began to prepare, mentally, for the big day: August 6. Egg Retrieval Day. Dr. Sahakian said I was ready. My eggs were juicy. It was time.

Ron and I both went into the clinic and they prepped me for the procedure. I was nervous, and I remember sitting on the table, trying to prolong the moment when they would put me under because after that, there would be no turning back, no more hoping. The eggs would be what they were. I talked and talked about this and that. I knew Dr. Sahakian had other people scheduled, but I couldn't stop myself. I sat there in my hospital gown asking questions about the eggs, the collapsed ovary, asking him to repeat everything he was going to do. He was very patient with me. I think I was trying to entertain them, too. I kept trying to pull them into my personal story, then makes jokes and crack them up. *If I make them laugh, they'll treat my eggs more carefully. They'll do the procedure better. I'll be more likely to get a baby.* It was like I was auditioning for a director. If I made them laugh or told them my deepest thoughts, I would have a greater chance of being cast in the role of "mother." I imagined the nurses whispering, "Doc, let's make sure the funny girl gets the baby!"

Egg retrieval requires anesthesia, so they put me out. While I was asleep, Ron had to do his part, giving them a good sample to use for the fertilization. I remember waking up in the office from the anesthesia and feeling calm and peaceful. It reminded me of waking up after an emergency appendectomy I'd had a few years back and feeling like everybody was taking care of me. I was drowsy when Dr. Sahakian came over and patted my wrist. His hand on my wrist felt like the best, most comforting thing in the world.

"That feels good," I said. "I'm very tired. I think I'll go back to sleep."

When I finally woke up, he told me I could get changed into my clothes and go. I didn't want to leave. I wanted to stay there, being cared for, while they made me a baby. When Ron and I walked out, I could hear another patient behind a curtain, although I couldn't see her or recognize her voice. It was the first time I'd ever seen anybody else in the office. They certainly were discreet.

Dr. Sahakian told me that he was able to retrieve eight viable eggs. Two were in excellent condition, three were pretty good, and three were average. The next step was to fertilize the eggs in the lab. I would come back in three days for the embryo transfer.

August 9, 2007, was Embryo Transfer Day, the day the doctor would implant the embryos and, we hoped, make me pregnant. It felt like a national holiday to me, but this was the day that Ron finally lost it.

He had misplaced a bag that contained his passport, and he was upset. Really upset. I knew the gravity of this moment—the moment I might become pregnant, I *would* become pregnant—so I began to snap at Ron for being upset about his passport. Who cares about a stupid passport when we're trying to make a baby here? Some part of me knew that the passport was just a trigger for the terrible stress we both felt about what might or might not happen in those moments after Dr. Sahakian worked his magic, but I couldn't verbalize this at the time. We poured all our anger, frustration, and fear into that passport argument, like it represented everything important about our future.

As we bickered, Dr. Sahakian kept reminding us that this should be a happy time, and that it was especially important not to be stressed because stress could make the procedure less likely to work. Still, we kept snapping at each other, and the air in the room got tenser and tenser as I got onto the tilt table, my head dangling toward the floor. I tried to breathe deeply and think calm, happy thoughts, but I was heartbroken as I lay there with my legs in the air. Then Doctor Sahakian inserted the embryos with a tool that looked like a turkey baster.

Happy thoughts, happy thoughts, happy thoughts . . . in went the embryos, and then I waited, still inverted, to increase the chances that the pregnancy would "take." Sweet music played in the air, as if I was in a spa, while the acupuncturist poked me with needles meant to relieve my fears and calm my stress. The acupuncture was meant to keep me in a peaceful state, so the embryo could implant. Upside down, a science experiment at its most crucial stage, I breathed deep, long, and full, *Think baby. Think happy. No stress.* Ha! It was one of the most stressful moments of my life! Sometimes I felt like I was married to Dr. Sahakian. He had all the information, all the power over my future status as a mother. He was the one inserting the embryos with a turkey baster. He was the only one who could make this happen for us.

So this was my impregnation? Lying on a steel table in a flimsy gown annoyed with Ron while a doctor inseminated me, overwhelmed with the fear that none of this was even going to work? The kindly nurse told me to relax, so I tried to relax into the whole bizarre scenario. It was the path we'd chosen, so it wasn't going to do any good to complain now. *Happy thoughts.* I felt ridiculous and unromantic. Even after they told me I could put my legs down and go home, I stayed. Just in case. I wanted to give my body every possible chance of success. Finally, after hours, Ron took me home. We were both exhausted, sorry, nervous. Hopeful, always hopeful.

Next came the waiting. I wouldn't know the answer for two weeks, but I didn't feel pregnant. I walked around like I was in a bubble, wondering, trying to feel something. I felt nothing. I was sure we would have to do it again.

On August 19, I went back for a blood test, and then I went home to await the results. I was told they would call me in the morning. It was the longest night of my life.

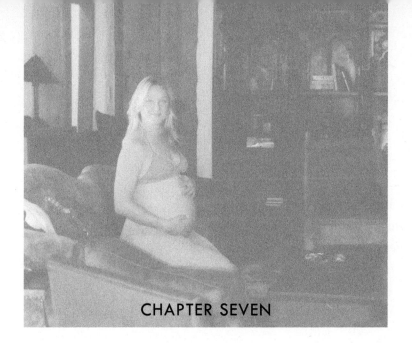

CHAPTER SEVEN

BODY

—

Why fit in when you were born to stand out?

—Dr. Seuss

and voluptuous bottom. I was never the five-foot-four waif who looked so charming next to the five-foot-ten leading man. I was the five-foot-ten actress who required a giant leading man—someone like Sam Waterston. I've been lucky enough to have those leading men who were six feet tall and more, but it wasn't always easy. I think, however, that I could handle it and that I didn't let it get to me at all, because of what my mother instilled in me from childhood: I've always had that foundational belief that I am beautiful exactly the way I am.

It's not just me. Yes, there is pressure to have a good body and look young and beautiful in Hollywood. Of course there is—it's part of the game. However, there are plenty of extremely successful women in Hollywood with real-world bodies, beautiful bodies, curvier bodies, bodies that aren't skinny but are real and sensual and lovely. Sure, sometimes I might overindulge and have a few second thoughts about whether I'll still look good when my show starts filming again, but then I just go back to the gym or go for a brisk walk or eat more vegetables. It's all good. Skinny is just one of a thousand ways to be beautiful. Hollywood is full of all kinds of beauty, just like the rest of the world, and having a unique look is often better for your career than looking like a Barbie doll. You have to be a little bit tough in the business, but I also believe there is room to be yourself, if you're brave enough to step in and take up that space.

So, thanks, Mom! I may not walk around naked in my house like you did, and when I change my clothes, I still close the bedroom door. But when my daughter does catch a glimpse of my body, she notices, and I see her internalizing her own ideas about the body. "Mommy, there's your butt! There's your boobs! There's your vagina! There's your back!"

Yes, Easton. Yes. It's my body, and it carried you, and bore you, and fed you, and thank God. I hug my daughter with this body. I cook food for her with this body. I love her father with this body. I get the extreme privilege of living my life every day in this body. I also notice that she has her own sense of modesty, and I love seeing her recognize what belongs to her and what is okay to show to the world. I love how she chooses to close the door when she changes, too, although I would also love her just as much if she chose to leave it open.

I remember saying to Dr. Sahakian, "I can't believe my body is broken," but I've come to learn, after all of this, that my body was never really broken. It was just unique, and it aged in a certain way that I didn't necessarily like, and it can't do everything I want it to do, but what body can? It has done what I needed it to do, even if it didn't always do it in the most perfect or expected way. I know now that this is enough for me.

We all have our body struggles—infertility, overweight or underweight, chronic diseases, whatever it is. For some of us, the burden of the body is much greater than for others, who may have other burdens: emotional, social, financial, familial. We also have our own unique shapes. I have small boobs and a big butt and a little bit of cellulite on the backs of my thighs. But you know what? I look at myself and I think, *Wow, you look damned good after taking all those fertility drugs and carrying a baby for nine months and being a working mom!* And I believe it.

IVF worked. I made it through pregnancy. I made it through childbirth. I breastfed blissfully. I still can't have another baby naturally, even though they say that sometimes, having a baby through IVF will kick-start the process and the next one just happens. So far, that hasn't happened for me, and if I want to have another baby, I'll have to do IVF again. And it might work. And it might not work.

But that's okay for now. I've found peace with my body.

Most importantly, I tell my daughter the same thing my mother told me: that *she* is beautiful, and her body is a treasure, and she should cherish it and honor and love it, no matter what it can or cannot do, no matter how it looks, no matter what anyone else says about it. I remind myself of the truth of these words every day, and I pray that my daughter will always believe them.

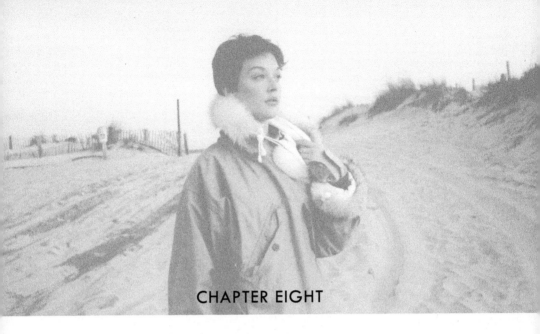

CHAPTER EIGHT

SECRETS

———

Three things cannot hide for long:
the moon, the sun, and the truth.
—**Herman Hesse**

*T*he Woodstock *I* know *might not be the* Woodstock *you imagine.* It's not a town full of tie-dye-clad groupies in a pot-induced haze refusing to admit it's no longer the 1970s. Okay, maybe it is a little bit like that, but it's also a small artist's community that my family and I call home. It's a place off the beaten path, a couple of hours from New York City, where we gather to be together in the beauty of upstate New York. To get there, I drive north through winding roads and miles of forest, literally removing myself from the frenetic and busy urban world. When I make that two-hour drive, I feel like I'm traveling deeper into my own life to get a closer, calmer look at myself.

Woodstock nurtures the free spirited. Artists flourish and live well here, making albums, writing books, painting, as they have for decades. It's a high-minded and open-hearted community. On any given day, you might drive through the humble little village and see people protesting against one of the wars or some other injustice on the village green. I'm not sure who they think will see them, but they protest nevertheless, because they believe it's the right thing to do, God love them!

Every time I go back there, I'm reminded that we all have a voice and we can all express ourselves in this country. And that's just what my family does, albeit in a less public mode. We gather at the home of my mom's best friend, Nancy, and we drink wine and eat amazing food because Nancy is a gourmet cook. And we talk. We talk about our lives and what is important to us. We relax. We let go of our work and our woes, and we exist there together in a happy bubble. We all feel comfortable in a town like Woodstock. A friend of mine once told me, "Lis, nobody knows who you really are. They think you are this shiny blonde with ice-blue eyes, and you're really just this crunchy hippie mama." To a family like mine, full of crunchy hippie types, Woodstock is heaven.

One evening a few years ago, a bunch of us sat around a table in Nancy's home eating her food and drinking her wine; Nancy's dinner parties are raucous and infamous, and everyone was in a good mood. I had been in New York City to meet with a director, and I couldn't go back to California without a visit to Woodstock, so there I was, with family and friends and Easton, only a few months old, asleep in the next room. I sat next to a distant relative I hadn't seen in a long time, and she had just congratulated me on my beautiful baby. Then her smile faded.

"I've had so many miscarriages," she said, her voice wavering. "Every time I get pregnant, I'm filled with so much hope, and then things start to go wrong. The last time . . ."

Everyone at the table fell silent. As she told her story, I realized many family members already knew. I hadn't visited in a while, so I was hearing about her troubles for the first time. Eight miscarriages.

I listened sympathetically, swallowing the urge to cry. Her eyes and her words were full of grief and longing and heartbreak, but I also remember feeling removed from what she was saying, in the way you might feel removed hearing someone talk about cancer or heart disease or losing someone in a car accident, if those things have never happened to you. I remember thinking, *I don't know what that's like.* I could sympathize with her. My heart ached for her and her husband, but because I couldn't relate personally, I really didn't know what to say.

As she talked, I sensed her hesitation. She was afraid of saying too much, or of not being able to continue. She was embarrassed. She was alone in front of us, even though the house was safe and she was in the heart of her family. The longer I listened, the more I wanted to rescue her. I felt uncomfortable sitting there listening with a blank expression on my face, as if I didn't really understand.

But I'd never had a miscarriage. What did I know about it?

And then I began to feel a familiar inkling, a recognition. Maybe I did know. She and I had both endured a great struggle in our quest to be mothers. We both knew grief and longing. Both our bodies had failed us. Both of us had been disappointed and disillusioned. Our stories were more similar than they seemed, even if the details differed. How dare I presume that I didn't know something about her pain! As I sat there nodding and smiling with compassion, I began to realize that I couldn't sit there acting like I knew nothing about what she was saying. How could I listen to another word and not tell her that my miracle baby had come out of a test tube? Why was I keeping it a secret?

I knew why. Ron and I had decided not to tell anyone. We wanted to celebrate the fairy tale of the pregnancy and the birth with our loved ones, rather than making it all about a medical problem. We were keeping it a secret, telling ourselves it was nobody's business, that it was a family matter, and that nobody had to know. I wondered what Ron would say if I told her. I wondered what she would think. I felt the same discomfort, at the prospect of telling my own secret, that I read in her face as she told hers, but I couldn't stand to see her standing in the middle of the classroom with her pants down. I wanted to stand up and say, "Okay, me too! Look, everyone! She's not so different!"

And yet, that discomfort, that embarrassment, held my tongue. Why? *Tell her, Lis,* I urged myself. *Tell her. Why not tell her?* Was my privacy worth so much that I couldn't throw her a lifeline? I couldn't comfort her? I couldn't tell her that I'd been frustrated and confused, too? And then, in a moment of clarity, in a sudden impulse of camaraderie, I said it:

"I completely understand." As I said it, I realized it was true. "I don't know what it's like to be pregnant over and over and have it taken away, but over the last two years, I've been battling infertility and I had to do IVF. Otherwise, I couldn't have had a baby."

She stared at me. "You did IVF?"

I nodded.

"To have Easton?"

"Yes." I swallowed and looked around at everyone.

She took my hand, and her sad face softened. "But you're so young!" she exclaimed.

And suddenly, we were on exactly the same page.

The most surprising thing about the whole experience was how relieved I felt, like a huge weight had been lifted from my shoulders. I told my secret to do something for her, and without realizing it, speaking it out loud had done something important for me. I felt different.

The things we keep secret, the things we don't say out loud, are really the things that we feel, at some level, are bad or wrong: what we do behind closed doors, or what has been done to us. The things we don't think other people will approve of. The things we think make us freaks, or inferior, or undesirable.

I didn't consciously think about infertility being "bad" until I spoke it that night. That's when I realized I had been ashamed of it all along. And then, when I said it out loud, I realized I didn't need to be ashamed of it anymore. It wasn't something I'd done wrong. And the more I began to talk about it, the more I realized how much I had suffered from the secret. When it wasn't a secret anymore, it was just something that was. It was just a truth.

Every woman has her secrets, and every woman has her own fertility story, whether it's the story of a pregnancy, or of trying to achieve a pregnancy, or of not realizing you wanted a baby, or of not being ready for a baby until it was too late. Sometimes, our fertility stories, our sexuality stories, and our self-worth stories get all tangled together and feel wrong and bad, and so we don't tell them. It becomes easy to forget how much all women have in common.

Some of us have stories of early menopausal changes (like mine), or of being unable to hold on to a pregnancy (like hers). Others have stories of losing the ones we love, or of enduring violence, or of medical issues we couldn't possibly control, but that nevertheless make us feel ashamed. Every woman's body tells a story, and whether or not you have been handed motherhood on a silver platter is all part of that story. When the stories of our bodies don't have happy endings, or even if they do have happy endings but only after a long hard struggle, it can feel like nobody knows what to say or how to help. It feels isolating and lonely, and it's easy to decide you are less than a "real" woman. When I tell other women about my story now, and I say that infertility can make you feel like you aren't a real woman, they nod their heads passionately, even if they haven't been through it. Every woman understands that fertility is intimately and deeply linked to being a woman, even for those who decide not to have children. When we *can't* do it the way we thought we could, we feel like less. We feel like freaks. We feel alone.

But it doesn't have to be that way. In particular, infertility doesn't have to be isolating. When someone else has been through it—when someone else takes your hand and says, "You know what? I get it because I've been through it, too, and it's a long road, I'm not going to lie, but if you ever want to talk about it, I'm here," well . . . those are powerful words.

I've kept some big secrets in my life, and I often didn't realize how much they were hurting me until I finally let them out. One of the biggest had nothing to do with infertility, but like many of the secrets women guard most ferociously, it had everything to do with my body.

When I was nineteen years old, I was in a nightclub in New York. I got myself into a situation that I couldn't get myself out of with a guy I barely knew. He was one of those people I sometimes ran into on the club scene, but as is the case with so many of those people you see while you are out partying and drinking, I only knew his first name. I'd been drinking that night, and I made some stupid decisions, and suddenly, there I was, being forced to do something I did not want to do and was not willing to do. When it was over, I pulled myself together and ran out of the club. It didn't occur to me to tell anyone or call the police—wouldn't it be his word against mine? I just had to get out of there. I had to remove myself from the situation as fast as possible, so I could forget it ever happened. He followed me into the street.

"Hey, do you need a ride home?" he said, as if nothing had happened. As if he hadn't just violated me. I couldn't even answer him. I shook my head.

He hesitated. "Okay. Well . . . do you have a headshot? Maybe I can help you out," he said. "In your career."

What? Really? I remember thinking that he must be trying to make up for what he'd just done to me, or somehow make it "fair." By boosting my career? Fuck him. I wanted to tell him to go to hell. I wanted to tell him, "You won't be seeing me ever again, just so you know, but thanks for the thought, asshole." But for some insane reason, I fumbled with my purse and pulled out one of my headshots and gave it to him. I don't know what I was thinking. It was an automatic response, or a survival response. *Just give him what he wants so you can get away,* I thought.

"Let me know if I can do anything!" he said, waving the picture in my direction.

"Okay," I said, turning away. I looked desperately for an escape route. Thank God, a cab. I jumped into the first one I saw, and I told the driver to take me to Bronxville, where I was going to college. As

soon as the driver pulled away from the club, I felt a huge sense of relief; I was fleeing the scene as if I'd been the perpetrator instead of
the victim. But I was so glad to put it all behind me. My body ached
and my head throbbed. I collapsed back into the seat, and then I realized I didn't have more than about three dollars in my purse. The
fifteen-miles-plus trip to Bronxville was going to cost a lot more than
three dollars. It was about four in the morning at the time, and for
some reason, right in the middle of Queens, I admitted to the cab
driver that I didn't have any money.

"As soon as you drop me off back at my dorm room, I'll run up and
get the money for you, I swear," I said. This was a bad idea. The cab
driver pulled into the first gas station and dropped me off. "You don't
have any money in your dorm room," he said. "Good luck, kid."

"Please! No, wait!" I pleaded. "I swear I'll pay you! I have money!"

He just shook his head and sped off to find a more lucrative fare.
And there I was, alone at a gas station in the middle of Queens in the
middle of the night. I turned around to get my bearings, and the first
thing I saw was yellow police tape around a chalk outline of a body
in the parking lot.

Oh my God, I thought. *Now I'm walking into a murder scene?* I began to imagine what else could happen to me. Would I make it home
alive? Terrified, I stumbled into a phone booth and frantically began
filling it with quarters, trying to get anyone I knew to answer the
phone. I practically screamed when someone rapped loudly on the
phone booth door. I whirled around. A man stood outside." Are you
okay?" he said.

I shook my head. I didn't know how to say yes at that point because it was so far from the truth.

"Do you want a ride somewhere?" he said. He gestured behind
him to a massive semi-tractor-trailer with a huge, cheerful Wonderbread logo on the side.

I hesitated. I was nervous to accept a ride from a stranger. It seemed like a rash and stupid thing to do, but I didn't see any other option at the moment. I nodded. I pushed open the phone booth door and he opened the front cab door for me. I climbed in, desperately rationalizing what I was doing. He was hauling Wonderbread. How dangerous could he be?

Just in case, I spent the whole ride trying to sound like the least sexy human being on the planet. I went for "nerd," talking about complicated books I'd read and referencing philosophers, hoping that would dampen any evil intentions, because at that moment, the whole world seemed threatening. He just nodded and answered benignly. "Uh-huh. Yep. Nope."

That truck driver, bless his heart, drove his giant Wonderbread semi all the way to Bronxville, right through my posh little college campus and into the driveway of the Tudor home that had been converted to a dormitory.

"Thank you so much," I said.

"My pleasure, ma'am," he said, before he backed up and piloted his lumbering vehicle back toward the interstate.

I went inside and went straight to bed. I didn't say anything to anyone. I swore I would take the secret with me to the grave. I would forget it ever happened.

And I did forget, for the most part, at least consciously, until a few years later.

When I was twenty-six years old, I received a book called *All About Me* as a gift. It was one of those books that contains questions you are meant to answer, and it gives you journal space to answer them. Questions like "What's the name of your mother?" "What's your favorite color?" "What are your regrets?" "What are you most proud of?" "If you had to be stranded on a desert island with one person, who would it be?" "What's your biggest secret?"

I've always loved things like this. When I was a teenager, I kept an adventure journal of all the things I'd ever done that I was proud of, like taking a train across the country, walking across the Brooklyn Bridge, and riding in a hot-air balloon. This book reminded me a little bit of my teenage adventure journal. I filled out all the pages, and when I came to the question "Tell the story of a secret you've never told anyone," I suddenly remembered that night in the nightclub when I was nineteen. I wrote about it in the book, with trembling hands and a quickening heartbeat. It was the first time I'd relived it, and part of me thought it might be good for me to write it down. Then I went on to the next question.

The week I finished filling out the entire book, Dick Wolf called and invited me to dinner. He had not yet cast me on *Law & Order*, but he had been my mentor since the *Invisible Man* pilot, and I was always hoping to be cast in his next venture. It occurred to me that I should bring along the *All About Me* book so he could see it. He had teenage children, and I know how teenagers tend to keep things to themselves. I thought he might like to see it and get something like it for them, to help them all communicate better. To create a conversation. I'd completely forgotten the details of what was written there.

We sat down at a table in a restaurant called The Palm on Santa Monica Boulevard, and I showed him my bright orange book. I told him how interesting it was to reflect so much on oneself. He began to flip through the book . . . and then he got to *that page*. The page where I'd told that secret. Only to myself. When I'd written it, I'd never imagined anyone else would read it. He paused on the page, his eyes scanning my words. Then he looked at me.

"Tell me about this," he said.

"Oh no!" I practically shouted, grabbing the book away. "I didn't want you to see that. I don't want to talk about *that*."

"Why not?" he said.

"I vowed to take that story to the grave with me," I said.

"Why?" he said.

I paused. Why? Why, indeed? I realized that I had always felt responsible for what happened to me that night. I'd been drinking. I put myself into an unsafe situation. I had taken the blame, which is why I never told a soul.

"I . . . don't want to remember," I said.

"Look, Lis," Dick Wolf said. "I'm in the process of creating a spin-off to *Law & Order* called *SVU*. It's about just this kind of thing. Everyone who is the victim of this kind of crime feels responsible and ashamed. They carry it around with them like an extra limb, hoping nobody sees it, even though it becomes part of who they are. I want people to be able to say, 'That happened to me,'" he said. "So it doesn't destroy them from within."

"Uh-huh," I said. I swallowed. It was like he'd read my mind.

"So tell me about it," he said. "Say it out loud."

Reluctantly, I told him the whole story.

"So, you were raped," he said.

I cringed at the word. I'd never spoken it in connection with what happened, even though he was right: that was what had happened. Deep down, I knew it was true. I nodded.

"Why don't you just say it out loud?" he said.

I bit my lip. It felt scary to say it, but what could it hurt? It already happened. Saying it wouldn't make it happen again. Maybe saying it would even help.

"I . . ." I paused. "I was raped," I said. The word hung there in the air between us. I wanted to take it back. I hated the way it sounded. But there it was.

"Did you say no to that guy?" he asked me.

"I did," I said. "More than once."

"Once, twice, a hundred times, it doesn't matter," he said. "No means no. It wasn't your fault. You were innocent."

In that moment, when I spoke my secret, and Dick Wolf told me I was innocent, I realized for the first time since it happened to me almost a decade ago that I *was* innocent. It didn't matter that I had been drinking. It didn't matter that I accidentally or carelessly put myself in an unsafe situation. It didn't matter that I never reported it, or never told anyone. I had done nothing to deserve it. I had not caused it. It wasn't my fault, and I didn't need to hold it inside me anymore. I could let it go.

I looked at him in amazement. I felt completely different, astounded that a secret from a decade before had actually become part of my personality, and now, just like that, it had evaporated, like darkness disappearing with the sun.

"Don't you feel better now that you said it out loud?" he said.

I did. I absolutely did.

"I wish I had known you back then," he told me. "I would have told you to take the bastard to court."

"Oh no, I wouldn't have wanted to do that!" I said.

Dick just shrugged. "I still would have encouraged it. But now you've told me, and you feel better. That's what I want for every person who's been a victim," he said.

Dick Wolf went on to create *Law & Order: SVU* to put a spotlight on sex crimes, and I know it's helped a lot of people. Maybe it's helped some to tell their stories and free themselves from the tyranny of the secret.

When it comes to infertility, this tyranny is no less real. This is the power that secrets have over us. The things we are most afraid to say

tended I didn't. You wanted me to have courage and confidence, and I do, Mom. I have all those things. Because of you. Every good thing I've ever done in my life, I've done because of you. I give you all the credit. You did it. You are the reason for my success. You did your job."

I waited, letting it sink in. I didn't want to say the next part, but I knew I had to say it. She needed to hear it. I knew she could hear me. I could feel it, that sense of her listening, waiting for my words, hovering over our two bodies. I didn't care what they said about brain activity. I wasn't speaking to her brain. I was speaking to her soul as it hovered over the bed, tethered to my heart.

"What I'm trying to say, Mom, is that it's okay for you to go. You're free now. You're free from this body, so you can fly away. Go to that place you've been waiting to see. God is ready for you. I'm going to be okay. Really. I'm going to be okay." Each time I said it, I believed it a little more.

I lay there for a long time after, and then suddenly, I felt like it was okay for me to go, too. I sat up stiffly and took her hand. "Good-bye, Mom. I love you. Thanks for being exactly the mom I needed." I kissed her hand and then I kissed her forehead, and then I stood up and walked out of the room without looking back.

After I left that hospital room, I asked Aunt Nancy if she would call the producers of *Heroes* and tell them that I wouldn't be coming back after the Thanksgiving break. I was just too exhausted to make the call myself. "I want to be here and help you clean the house and I want to be here when she . . . when she goes," I said, swallowing. "I want to be here for everything."

Nancy shook her head. "She would want you to go back to work," she said. "She was so incredibly proud of you. She wouldn't want to be the reason for you giving up anything good in your life. And most importantly, she would want you to go home and take care of Easton."

I didn't like the way she was already speaking of my mom in the past tense, even though I understood that in so many ways, my mother was already gone. "But I don't want to leave," I said. "I want to be here when she passes. It's important for both me and Mom."

"Even if she wouldn't want that?" Nancy pressed.

I looked at the sterile floor of the hospital. I knew that maybe she was right. Maybe my mother, despite my words to her, wouldn't go until I left. I called my Aunt Laurie and after a long discussion, she encouraged me to go home, too, for Easton's sake.

And so I packed, and got into the car, and drove to the Amsterdam airport, and got on a plane, knowing my mother's heart was still beating. When I arrived at the London airport, I called Nancy. My mother had passed away forty-five minutes after I left Amsterdam.

Maybe this sounds like a neat little picture, the perfect romantically tragic ending, but I didn't feel that way at all. I could have told myself that she needed me to leave in order to be free, but I didn't really believe it. It broke my heart that she was gone, and I didn't know for sure if I should have left at all. I was filled with doubt and regret. What if she wanted me to be there, and I abandoned her right at the last minute? I couldn't let the feelings go. I had no resolution because I wasn't there to see her go. I tortured myself with the question, *Was she waiting for me to leave, or did I leave too soon?* When she took her last breath, was her spirit looking for me, and I wasn't there? If I had stayed, would I have had more closure? Would she have come back awake? Everybody kept telling me to let her go, and I had to make a decision for the whole family, right at the moment when I was the least clear and least able to do the sensible thing. That tore me apart for months.

I went back to Los Angeles newly initiated to the cold terror of being a motherless child. I was thirty-six years old but I felt like an orphan.

Do I wish she had stayed on life support for months, even years, until it was confirmed to me without a doubt that the doctors were right and I was wrong, until I had time to get used to the idea of her passing, until I had time to really feel like I had said good-bye? Yes. I do wish for all those things, whether I should or not. I feel like she was ripped away from me, unjustly and cruelly. I felt like she was cheated out of the pleasures of becoming a wise old woman, cheated out of seeing her granddaughter grow up to be a woman herself.

When I went back to *Heroes*, I was a different person than the person who left. On *Heroes*, I played a character called Lauren Gilmore, who worked with the character Noah Bennett, played by Jack Coleman. Jack and I played business partners and romantic interests, so we had become friends, and thank goodness for Jack. Jack had lost his mother, and I knew this, so he was the only one I told about where I was going, and as soon as I got back to the set, he could tell by looking at me that my mother was gone.

He was a source of compassion on the set, when nobody else knew what had happened. I didn't want them to know. I wasn't ready to talk about it. I didn't want anyone to ask me if I was okay (because I was *not* okay) and I didn't want to see pity in their faces. Why tell everybody? But knowing that Jack knew gave me some peace. When he looked at me, it wasn't with pity. It was with a look that said, "You're going to be okay because I'm here and I'm standing and I'm okay." Eventually, I was able to tell others, as I got used to saying the words: "My mother has died."

This was in the fourth season of *Heroes*, and we were filming the final three episodes. There were rumors that the show wouldn't be renewed, so the cast was connected and intensely focused on making the final three episodes as amazing and effective as we could, hoping it would keep the show afloat. *Heroes* was a show about the meaning of life, and the people on the outskirts looking in. It was about the conflicts between right and wrong and love any loyalty. Lauren and Noah were out to take down and destroy something they didn't understand, and Noah was conflicted because his own daughter (played by Hayden Panettiere) was part of what he didn't understand. My character was also trying to do her job; like Serena Southerlyn, she was bound by law, and yet, the passionate part of her wanted to break the rules in the name of love. In the end, on the show, love becomes more important than what is right.

I believe that to be true in my own life, too—in my relationships with my mother, my daughter, the man I love, even with my friends. Love is more important than what is right. I think about this when I think about my mother because she didn't always do what was "right." Should she have sent me away to boarding school at fourteen? Should she have sold our childhood house to pursue her strange and unique dreams? Should she have torn up that Social Security card? Should she have walked around the house naked? Should she have told me all about her money problems, her spiritual conflicts, her every emotional bump in the road? Should she have given up everything for me, and should she then have taken it all back to go find herself?

Yes. Yes, yes, yes, because it was all for love—love for me, for herself, love for God, and a great passionate love for life.

My little family recently moved out of the house we'd lived in since my daughter was born, and that event was just one of thousands that made me realize that nobody but a mother wants to hear the blow-by-blow details of your everyday existence. Of course I could talk to my friends, but honestly, nobody but your mother cares if you are moving. Nobody really wants to hear about it. Nobody wants to help. If my mother had been there, she would have wanted to hear every detail. *How's the light? How's the water pressure? Describe the kitchen.*

Did you check for mildew? Send Easton to my house while you move. I'll take care of everything.

I long for those days when she would call me at 6:00 A.M. to hear everything about my life. I can't forget that conversation when I told her we should table our early-morning chats for a while, because I wanted to focus on myself. I think about every word, every sentence I didn't get to hear from her or say to her. All lost. She understood the need for solitude better than anyone, but I still regret my withdrawal from her. I would give almost anything to hear that phone ring. I would answer it with joy and gratitude and I would talk to her up until the last second when I absolutely had to hang up and get to work. I would tell her every single detail, no matter how trivial: what I had for lunch, every syllable my daughter speaks, what the dog did, how the weather is, all about my latest acting project, why the new house really was better than the old house, what I would miss about the old house, and how bittersweet it is to move on from the things you love. I'm greedy for every lost moment. I want them all back.

Instead, I have these conversations with myself, unmoored as I am now from the grounding force and anchor that was her. She wanted me to love something beyond this world, and oh how I do. Mom, where are you now? What's it like? How's the light? Are you finally free? Can you feel how much love I'm sending out into the ether? Does it find you?

Because she was still alive when I last saw her, sometimes I feel like she's still out there somewhere, living out the rest of her life, the decades she should have remaining. She cannot answer me, not yet, but I'll never stop asking. She wanted me to keep seeking, and I do— I seek God, I seek love, I seek *her*. Because my mother is gone from this world.

Her gifts were not lost on me and that is my one consolation. I see how she created me in her own image, and how she also created me in the image of myself, so that I could become someone who had never existed before and will never exist again. She made me see my own beauty and uniqueness. She taught me that what I need matters more than what society thinks I should want. It was her legacy. My mother didn't do everything right, but she got the big things right. The soul-oriented, character-creating things were what mattered to her, and I can only hope I can be half the mother she was.

My mother was strong and passionate and she walked this earth with a power all her own, and she bestowed it on me. To be a mother is, in some sense, to be supernatural. To be full of magic. To be eternal. To understand at the level of soul that love is more important than what is right, and to act on that—to love through fear and pain and even through death.

That is why she was, and is, and always will be my hero.

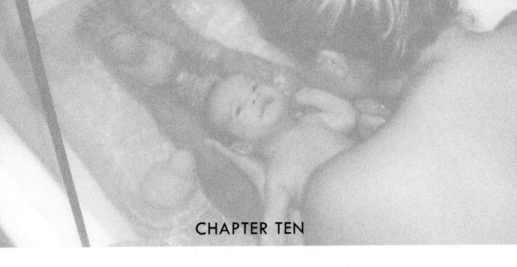

CHAPTER TEN

MIRACLES

The world is so rich,
simply throbbing with rich treasure.
—Henry Miller

The first time I felt the miracle of pregnancy wasn't when I heard my baby's heartbeat or saw her on the ultrasound monitor. It was the moment when I first felt her move inside me.

Ron and I were visiting Turks and Caicos along with some other celebrities for the opening of a beautiful new hotel. The hotel was promoting itself and invited us, and I was looking forward to a relaxing weekend in the Caribbean. The hotel was beautiful—bright yellow with white hurricane shutters, decorated in pastels and infused with the aroma of patchouli and gardenias. In the airport, I recognized Giuliana Rancic and her husband, and although we didn't really know each other, we waved. (I wish I had known then what I know now—she could have ordered up a stiff drink and I could have ordered a virgin piña colada and we could have swapped infertility stories!)

I was about six and a half months pregnant at the time. After we checked into the hotel, I looked out at the vast turquoise ocean and told Ron I was going to go swimming. I put on my maternity bathing suit and went down to the beach. I waded into the warm water and lay back to float. I wanted to get some exercise, so I paddled around gently on my back. Suddenly, I felt the baby roll over!

Oh my God! I looked down at my swollen belly and I saw her foot or her hand pressing out toward me, reaching out to me. I touched it, and I felt like we held on to each other for the first time. I waded back out and went back up to the room to show Ron. She was still moving. He put his hand on my belly and she kicked and turned for him, too. He looked at me in wonderment. It was a miracle. I was growing a life inside me. For the first time, it felt real.

Life is full of little miracles like this. When I look back over my life, I can think of a lot of examples of people showing up and reminding me who I am or where I am or what I really want to be doing, just at the moment when I could have gone in the wrong direction or forgotten what was important. It might be a random taxi driver in New York saying something out of the blue that helps me keep my head on straight. It might be a server in a diner or my agent or manager or lawyer, or it might be my Aunt Laurie or Ron or even my daughter. I think God speaks through people sometimes, in order to tell you what you need to hear. Words that seem to come from the beyond have often helped me to find my way again. I think that anyone with eyes wide open is likely to run smack into all kinds of miracles in this life. You just have to pay attention.

Having a baby was my greatest miracle, but after my mother died, my miracles began to come hard and fast. When she was alive, calling me every day from Amsterdam, she would sometimes say, "I'm so frustrated that I can't help you. I can't help you with finances because I don't have any money. I can't help you with child care because I'm not in the best of health. I can't help you by being there because I'm an ocean away." One day, she said, "I would be more help to you if I was in heaven!"

After she died, I was practically laid out by grief, and after *Heroes* ended, I was feeling a lot of career and financial pressure. Then, out of nowhere, I was cast in a movie I'd been interested in a year before, but that I thought was never going to be made. The best thing about the movie was that it would be filming in New Jersey, so I was able to go back home to New York and stay at Nancy's house in Scarsdale. I could bring Easton, and I would have the family support and help I needed. It was a dream come true at that moment in my life.

Shortly after filming the movie, I was called back to New York again to make a two-hour personal appearance at an event for animals. The honorarium seemed disproportionately large. All I had to do was go to a party and give a speech in a ballroom full of pets and pet lovers about my love for animals. It was amazing. It was something I was more than happy to do, and I felt like the money had fallen from the heavens.

I just know she choreographed all of it. She was sending me the help I needed. The child care help, the career boost, the financial boost, and the family support I craved. After that, I got another starring role in a studio film called *Transit*, opposite Jim Caviezel, an actor with a strong sense of spirituality. Of course, my mother, from her heavenly vantage point, would put me into a film with someone like that. Then, other miracles: I began to write a blog at People.com, and then through a series of coincidences, I met the writer who could help me with this book. And now I'm writing it! It all seems so unlikely, so beautiful, and so perfectly orchestrated. I cannot believe it was all coincidence.

Then, last December, I was praying to God that I didn't want to travel so much anymore because I wanted to be home more often with my daughter, so she could have more stability and be able to count on my being there every day. I prayed, "God, please keep me at home unless travel really enhances our lives. I want to work in LA." Very soon after that, I began to notice a couple at my daughter's school. I'm not sure why I noticed them, but when I saw them in Whole Foods one afternoon, I went up to them and said, "For some reason, I feel like I'm supposed to know you."

They both said they felt the same way, even though none of us knew why connecting suddenly seemed important. I had no idea that one of them was a screenwriter and a director. After two or three playdates, she said, "I've heard through the grapevine that they are casting a new show called *The Client List* with Jennifer Love Hewitt and they are looking for a character that would be the perfect fit for you. Have your agent set up a meeting." Before I knew it, I had the part—a television show based in Los Angeles. It was just what I'd asked for. I'm working, playing a part I enjoy, and I'm right here for my daughter.

I've spent most of my life on a quest for God, following in my mother's footsteps. Every moment of my childhood was deeply tie-dyed with my mother's spiritual quest, and I never went through that stage of rejecting religion or spirituality, like some kids do. I always assumed and knew this was part of what it means to be alive in a human body—we are always seeking something more than we can see and touch.

This is probably why I'm so open to the idea of miracles. I was baptized as a Christian and went to an Episcopalian boarding school. I sang in the church choir, but I also spent my summers and many a weekend with my mother at ashrams, wearing saris and meditating and talking about Buddhism, Hinduism, and other Eastern-influenced concepts. When my mother was a devotee of Gurumayi and we spent extended periods at her opulent ashram in New York, I felt at home.

The summer of my sixteenth year, Gurumayi herself noticed me in a crowd of other kids. She had her swamis talk to me, and one thing led to another, until I became part of her entourage, one of the kids who participated in the ceremonies. I wore saris on all the high holidays and Gurumayi even gave me an Indian name, a spiritual name. She hadn't given my mother a spiritual name. When Gurumayi asked me to accompany her to India, I seriously considered it. It was flattering and made me feel special to be one of her "chosen ones." But after thinking long and hard about it, and talking to my mother about it, I decided it was more important for me to finish high school, so I went back to my boarding school in Tennessee after the summer was over.

Still, it all made a great impression on me, and I've continued to be spiritually engaged. I don't really subscribe to any "ism." Instead, my religion is about living a conscious life, being kind and simple in the way I was raised to be. By the time I got to college, I was so versed in world religions that it was no longer about religion but about a quest for God. Miracles seem self-evident to me, and I believe this is because of my mother. She always said that I could believe whatever I wanted to believe, as long as I accepted what others believed. She wanted me to be tolerant and educated, and at the same time, open to the shifting energies of spirit, the idea of faith, and the wonders of a universe we barely comprehend in our limited human form. I have all of that inside me because of her. She was my biggest spiritual influence.

When you stay open to possibility, anything might happen. I really believe that. You don't necessarily need to know what's going to be right for you. Life is about staying awake and aware and keeping your options open, and this notion helped me through my battle with infertility. There are so many possibilities for every life, and so many ways to be a mother, and so many little people out there who need a mother's love and, I believe, so many souls waiting to come down into a body on this earth to love and be loved. Maybe one of them has already picked you out.

When my daughter was two years old and just beginning to talk well, she told me, "I saw you down there, Mama, walking around."

"What?" I said. "Where did you see me? When?"

"Before," she said simply. "I saw you down there."

From where? From heaven? From some other realm? Before she was born? She couldn't tell me any more, but I think I know. I'm not a crazy person, but I think my daughter's soul knew exactly where it was going, before it took that plunge into the earthly realm. There is so much more to life than what we currently know or understand. Ron and I always call her our miracle baby, and this was just one more bit of evidence that indeed she is, and that she chose us. It was a miracle that she found me down here, but somehow, she did.

For as many times as things have been challenging, there have been many more times when things have been right: the fact that I found Ron, that I had my miracle baby, that I had so many surprising opportunities in my career, that I found the grace and inner strength to forgive my parents, and that that they have forgiven me my trespasses, too. Forgiveness is always a miracle, and all four of my parents have enacted their own miracles in my life.

It wasn't a miracle that I have fertility issues. That sucks. But it was a miracle that I went to Cambodia, that I found Dr. Sahakian, and that IVF worked on the first try. It is a miracle that I live in a time and place and circumstance in which I have IVF available to me. It was a miracle that my mother lived long enough to meet my daughter, and that my daughter came to me and that she is exactly the person she needs to be.

I could name a thousand miracles in my life. A hundred thousand. When I think back, I see that it's all been a miracle, the natural order of things playing out, and how people show up and events happen just when you need them. I used to think the phrase "When a door closes, another one opens" was such bullshit, until I experienced the truth of it myself. Everything works out as it should, if only you're willing to see it that way. You just have to get out of your own way and stop assuming your own defeat. There will still be defeats in every life—but there can also be greatness in their wake.

In my mind, the miracles in my life are not just things that happened. They are something more: the shifting, breathing conscious machinations of Spirit—the light or God or energy or hand of fate that knows me and brings me what I need, and what I most purely and passionately desire. I believe miracles are divine interventions that help to keep me on a divine path. I think they are orchestrated, and I believe they are available to anyone willing to see them and act accordingly. It's easy to feel like your prayers aren't being heard. Oh

At seven months, my milk dried up and I was heartbroken to give up breastfeeding. For two years, I was profoundly exhausted. But in the best possible way, I had *changed*. I suddenly had a real purpose, and a love bigger than any I'd ever experienced. I think I must have become more interesting to everyone around me. I also felt like I was healing from every childhood injury I'd ever experienced.

I began to see how desperately I had always tried to deal with the shadows of my past, to repair my own pathology, and then suddenly, this thing that happened to me, this becoming a mother with a baby, it lifted me effortlessly out of my obsession with my own life.

I began to feel happy.

I had always been so focused on how to be happy despite my past. I had always blamed my parents. But when I held my baby in my arms, late at night, rocking slowly back and forth in the nursery while gazing through the blinds at the moonlight and listening to the sounds of the night, I realized that happiness doesn't come from looking at yourself. It comes from looking toward others.

I'd always wanted to be a good person, to be kind, to give to others, and I'd always wanted to feel better about myself, but when I had Easton, all I wanted was to be strong, to be powerful, to be an artist, and to fight for everything I've earned because *she* deserved a mother who knows who she is and knows how to make home a happy place.

"You deserve to be happy," my mother would tell me in those early weeks, when she got up with the baby sometimes, so I could get some rare and wonderful sleep. My mother told me I was a natural. She told me I was a good mom, and it was the greatest compliment anyone could have ever given me. "Now you know how to love," she said. "I know you've struggled through your life. I know you've been angry about your childhood, about your dad leaving, about having to go to that school, about a lot of things. Maybe now you don't have to be angry anymore. Maybe now you understand love in a different way."

I don't mean to make it sound like everything in my life was fixed. It wasn't. Nobody tells you that love is hard, that you're going to get your heart broken, that the things you want the most might not come to you as easily as you hope. Nobody tells you how difficult it is to be a parent. And nobody tells you that a baby doesn't solve all your problems, especially if you struggle with infertility. You probably wouldn't believe them if they did. But I'll tell you. A baby is a miracle, a wondrous gift, but a baby is not a panacea. It doesn't make you into somebody you never were. It doesn't make you a different person. You're still the same person, with all the same faults, but a baby can help you to become okay with your faults. A child doesn't cure you, but it can heal you.

Here's the truth. When you have a baby, when you finally get the thing you've wanted more than anything else, you might still feel depressed sometimes, or anxious, or unhappy. Sometimes you're going to wish for your freedom. Sometimes you're going to want to run away. Sometimes you're going to put your head into your hands and sob because it all seems like too much to bear and all you really want is a couple of hours of sleep.

I realize all this now, but nevertheless, having a baby was the best thing I ever did. Yes, sometimes I still want to run away. I want to shut myself in the bathroom with a bottle of chardonnay and pretend nobody is ever going to ask me to do anything for them ever again. I love Easton with all my heart, but that doesn't mean she's not going to throw a tantrum or demand something she can't have or tell me that she doesn't like me, even if, two minutes later, she climbs into my lap and nestles against my chest like a little kitten.

The other day, she told me I was a bad mommy because I was ignoring her. I was reading a script at home in the afternoon.

"But Easton," I said. "I'm here all day with you. I just have to do a little work."

"I don't care," she said. "I want a new mommy who will play with me all day."

Nobody tells you that your baby is going to break your heart, a thousand times a day—when she won't stop crying and won't be comforted by you, when she turns toward someone else with a delighted smile, when she doesn't need you to help her with something anymore. A baby can break your heart just by gazing at you with all the love her soul contains, by reaching for you to pick her up, or by smiling at you for the first time. The first belly laugh, the first surprised expression at the first bite of real food, the first tooth coming in or falling out, the first Halloween costume, the first Easter, the first day of school—they are all heartbreakers.

She will break your heart when she takes her very first steps in the opposite direction, away from you. Because that's where she's headed. Nobody tells you that.

When I was a little girl, my mother often said to me, "You're my greatest teacher." She always wanted my opinion, even when she started dating again. "Do you like him? You have great intuition. You always know the answer. What do you think?" she would ask me.

This made me feel smart, but as I grew up, I began to suspect that I wasn't her greatest teacher after all. How could I be? She was an adult, and she was *my* greatest teacher. What did I know, a mere child? What could I possibly teach her? She was just trying to build my confidence. She was trying to make me feel important.

Then I had a daughter. Now, I realize that my mother was telling me the truth, as was her way. I know I was her greatest teacher, because my daughter has become *my* greatest teacher. She tests me every day, the way I tested my mother. She loves me unconditionally because it is part of her biology; not because we are related, but because I am the one who has always hovered over her, fed her, clothed her, rocked her to sleep, soothed her cries, come to her room in the middle of the night, read her stories, and held her hand.

She makes me a better person. She keeps me on my toes. She challenges me to be my best, especially when she's at her worst. She reminds me that she is only at her worst when she needs me the most.

That's what my mother meant.

About eight months before my mother died, we had a sort of impromptu family reunion at Nancy's house in Woodstock. It was the spring of 2009, and it was our birthday month, Easton's and mine. Easton was just about to turn one.

Nancy's home was the perfect place for us to meet. It was a home full of happy memories, about halfway between Los Angeles, where I was coming from, and Amsterdam, where my mother was coming from. It was the place where Nancy married Olaf, and my mother met Peter. It was the place where we had all spent so many happy times over the years. It was a place of rebirths—new love, rekindled relationships, and family.

The evening everyone arrived, the house was full of laughter and mirth. Everyone was there. Ron and Easton and I, my mother and Peter, who brought his pickled herring from Europe, Nancy and Olaf, Olaf's children, and all the friends who lived nearby. It was a revolving door of loved ones. The red wine was flowing and the house was full of wonderful food, thanks to Nancy. We had all my favorite dishes: olives and cheese, mushroom risotto and arugula salad, and my favorite birthday cake, flourless chocolate.

Everything was perfect. Nancy lives on an acreage with trees and fields and chickens, and the house is rustic and eclectic, with long wooden benches in the dining room, a stone fireplace, glass coffee tables and elegant furniture, and a vast picture window that looks out onto the fields and the huge sky and the flower garden my mother planted for Nancy every year. Behind the house, trees covered in pink petals fluttered beneath rustling pines, and at night we could hear birds and frogs and the gentle buzz of insects drifting in through the open windows.

The best part about that night was watching my mom with Easton. I wanted so desperately for them to know each other, even though my mother lived so far away. I hungrily watched as my mom delighted in every little thing Easton did: the way she ate her baby food, the cute little almost-talking noises she made, the way she kept trying to take her first steps, grasping onto the edge of the glass coffee table and bouncing up and down on her chubby little legs. My mom sat on the floor with Easton to play with her and read her books, even though I know this was hard for her.

I have a photograph from that night, of my mother sitting in a chair. I'm sitting on the floor in front of her. My mother is massaging my back and I'm cuddling Easton. It's a live snapshot in my mind: three generations, physically intimate, emotionally engaged, spiritually connected.

"I want to see you *ten* times a year," I complained to my mom that night. "Not just two or three."

"Let's do that," she said. "Let's both make sure we do that. We'll go back and forth more often. I'll come here to help you, and you'll bring Easton to Amsterdam."

"We will!" I said, with such conviction, even though our next visit wasn't planned until Christmas, when my mother would come to California. She wouldn't live long enough to make that trip.

But I didn't see the future. I lived in the beautiful present moments of that week in Woodstock. My mom wanted as much time with Easton as she could get, so she kept shooing me away to go for a run or get some time to myself. I remember thinking, *This is what family is for. This is how it's supposed to be, all of us raising a child together, supporting each other.*

On the last night of our visit, my mother decided she was going to teach Easton to walk, even though she'd recently had two hip replacements and walked with a cane. She seemed frail to me. Her health was failing more than I knew.

Easton had spent the whole week scooting everywhere, holding on to things, trying to pull herself up, crawling up the stairs, really moving. My mom had spent the week following her, shadowing her, being on call while I relaxed. That night, in front of a roaring fire, my mother took Easton's hands. Easton stood up. Everyone in the room fell silent.

We all watched as Grammy and Baby stepped slowly, slowly across the room, one unsteady woman and one unsteady baby making their way together. My mother seemed livelier than she had all week. Suddenly she let go and stepped back and I held my breath. Easton looked startled for a moment, then her eyes fixed on my mother and she became determined. With one little foot, and then the other, haltingly, but bravely, she stepped out on her own and half waddled, half tumbled the four feet into my mother's waiting arms.

Everyone cheered. I felt like the luckiest woman on the planet.

It was the last day my mother was ever present with me, the last time I touched her skin while she was conscious, the last day we spoke to each other. It was a good day, full of love and hope for the future of our family. She told me one last time that day that I deserved to be happy. And I was.

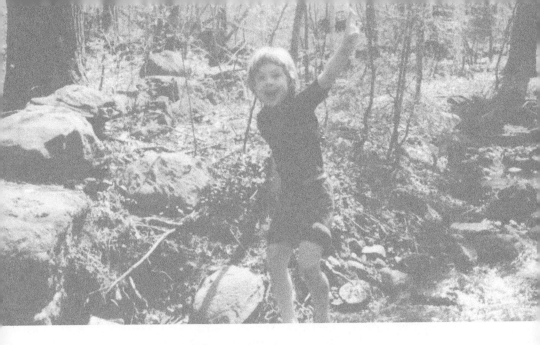

EPILOGUE

_Children are the living message we send
to a time we will not see._

—John W. Whitehead

If I could build a new world, I would make it a world where everyone who wanted a child could have a child, and everyone around that child would join together to raise it into a strong, courageous, loving human being. Gender wouldn't matter. Sexual orientation wouldn't matter. Money wouldn't matter. Age wouldn't matter. Anyone with love to spare could raise a child, and we would all be there to help that child take her first steps across a room filled with family and friends.

If I could build a new world, I would make sure every woman in her early twenties starts thinking about when she wants to have a baby and gets ready, just in case. In my new world, the older women who are so beautiful in their experience and maturity would be just as ready to conceive as the young woman just growing into herself. In my world, everyone who wanted to give birth to her own baby could do so easily and naturally.

In this new world, all parents would devote their lives to their children, and whole communities would rise up to help, and all children would grow up to be good parents themselves, and everyone would feel a deep and abiding sense of belonging. When things went wrong, as they inevitably do, people would speak up and reach out to each other and say what really matters: "I hurt. I need you. I can't do it alone. I'm overflowing with love."

Family comes in many forms, but it is always a mirror. Family shows us who we are, what we're made of. It proves our ability to love, even under the most trying circumstances. Ideally, family lifts us up. It is the source of our lowest and highest moments. It is the scaffolding on which we hang our hearts. It is love incarnate, and when a baby comes, the love expands and expands until it encompasses everything. The ones we love are our greatest teachers.

So I propose we expand our definition of family, and our requirements for the dispensing of our affection. I propose that we move toward this new world, because this world could be *our world,* if only we would all decide such a world of acceptance, tolerance, honesty, and community was worth having. There is space for everyone. Let's open our arms.

I have many more adventures ahead of me. My daughter is only four years old. I may or may not try to have another child. I may or may not walk down the aisle. I may or may not walk *her* down the aisle someday. I won't live forever, and neither will she.

But as long as I still walk on this earth, I will fight for a world that champions all versions of family. Let's say what we feel. Let's do what we need to do. Let's listen, and reach out, and help, and hold each other up, and stop letting each other down. Let's speak up and support anyone who wants to love a child, without making them feel ashamed or wrong or broken. I believe we can make that happen. I believe it's already beginning. I see it every day. One by one, women are standing up, raising their hands, and saying, "I can't have a baby the 'regular' way, but I still want to have a baby!"

Yes, the world is big, and full, and it doesn't always seem like the best place for a child. Life is hard and the world spins through the light and through the dark, and we don't always know what's going to happen to us next. Sometimes, things don't work out the way we thought they would. But they do work out, one way or another.

If you have love to give to a child, then I say give it. Any way you can. Give it all away.

LETTER FROM DR. SAHAKIAN

I first saw Elisabeth Rohm in July of 2007, when she was thirty-four. At the time, she had been trying to conceive for about a year and a half, and had been unsuccessful. She struck me as a beautiful and strong woman who was determined not to waste any more time, and I found this incredibly refreshing. She was not afraid to make tough decisions and follow through with them.

Elisabeth's determination to act quickly was unusual. Most women at her age procrastinate when it comes to fertility problems, often until it's too late. They don't realize how much age affects fertility. Most women think that if they are healthy, they exercise, and they look great, then having a baby will be easy. This is far from the truth! Unfortunately, even some ob-gyns take age lightly and don't stress the urgency to their patients.

Infertility can become a problem decades before menopause occurs, and women don't always understand this. In many cases, the cause is something called accelerated ovarian aging. For unknown reasons, in cases of accelerated ovarian aging, eggs are prematurely lost and quality deteriorates faster than expected. For example, the ovaries of a thirty-four-year-old woman might behave as if they are forty years old. This translates to lower pregnancy rates and therefore the urgency. You won't know if you have this problem unless you test your ovarian reserve. If you do have it and you want to have a baby, you will likely need to seek aggressive treatment, the way Elisabeth did. You never know whether this could happen to you. Elisabeth didn't know. There were no other symptoms.

As far as treatment is concerned, IVF (in vitro fertilization) is the best treatment for age-related decline in fecundity. The concept is simple. If the problem is that you have lower-quality eggs due to aging, then the only way to compensate for that decline in quality is by increasing quantity. IVF offers you the ability to do exactly that. Doing an IVF cycle is the equivalent of trying on your own for several months, so you are basically condensing time into a single month of treatment. It speeds up time, just when you have no time to lose.

What I hope this book accomplishes is to send out a message to all women that when it comes to fertility, age matters and time is a woman's worst enemy. I can do a lot of magic, but I cannot turn back the clock. Women are born with a set number of eggs that they use during their reproductive years. By the time a woman is fifty or fifty-one, her eggs have run out and menopause ensues. Unfortunately, before that last egg disappears, the eggs a woman has left tend to deteriorate genetically.

Many people consider infertility a taboo. Women are ashamed to admit that they are infertile, as if infertility somehow makes them less womanly. Of course this isn't true, and it's a shame that people feel this way, because the secrecy surrounding infertility and IVF plays a big role in keeping this topic away from general knowledge. It propagates the ignorance that's out there regarding age and infertility. Many well-known public figures who have used IVF to conceive not only keep it a secret, but actually pretend that they conceived naturally. Unfortunately, this causes more harm than good, as it gives false hope to women who think that if a celebrity got pregnant at forty-five, then so can they.

What Elisabeth is doing by writing her memoirs and revealing her experience with infertility and the fact that she had to do IVF to con-